The Institute of Biology's
Studies in Biology no. 141

Nutrition and Health

T. Geoffrey Taylor
M.A., Ph.D., F.I.Biol.
Rank Professor of Applied Nutrition,
University of Southampton

Edward Arnold

First published 1982
by Edward Arnold (Publishers) Limited
41 Bedford Square, London WC1 3DQ

British Library Cataloguing in Publication Data

Taylor, T. Geoffrey
   Nutrition and health. – (The Institute of Biology's studies in biology, ISSN 0537; no 141)
   1. Nutrition
   I. Title   II. Series
   613.2   TX353

ISBN 0-7131-2840-2

Photoset and printed by Photobooks (Bristol) Ltd
Barton Manor, St. Philips, Bristol 2

General Preface to the Series

Because it is no longer possible for one textbook to cover the whole field of biology while remaining sufficiently up to date, the Institute of Biology proposed this series so that teachers and students can learn about significant developments. The enthusiastic acceptance of 'Studies in Biology' shows that the books are providing authoritative views of biological topics.

The features of the series include the attention given to methods, the selected list of books for further reading and, wherever possible, suggestions for practical work.

Readers' comments will be welcomed by the Education Officer of the Institute.

1982

Institute of Biology
41 Queen's Gate
London SW7 5HU

Preface

This book is a sequel to book no. 94 in this series, *Principles of Human Nutrition*. The earlier book was mainly concerned with theoretical aspects of nutrition whereas the present one is devoted to more practical matters and it assumes a knowledge of basic principles. Thus, for example, the concept of protein quality is not defined and it is assumed that the reader knows what fats, carbohydrates, minerals and vitamins are. Only in this way was it possible to maximize the amount of new material that could be included.

The central theme of the book is 'Nutrition and Health' and the aim throughout is to give an up to date account of this relationship and, on the other side of the coin, of the relationship between nutrition and some important disease conditions. All too many nutritionists in their popular writings attribute excessive importance to individual nutrients such as sugar, fat or fibre, for example, thereby confusing the public and ignoring the first principle of nutrition which is that all nutrients are important and all must be balanced with respect to one another. This book attempts to present a balanced view of particular areas of nutrition, selected on the basis of their importance to health.

Southampton, 1982   T. G. T.

Contents

1 General Aspects of Nutrition and Health

1.1 Introduction

The link between nutrition and health is generally accepted and this link is most clearly demonstrable in cases of extreme under- or over-nutrition, examples of which are considered in Chapters 2 and 3 respectively. The term *malnutrition* embraces both under- and over-nutrition and there is a range of intake of individual nutrients and of energy in between these two extreme situations, narrow for some nutrients, wider for others, which promotes a state of optimum nutrition. The concept of optimum *ranges* of intake is important and it carries the implication that the body is able to compensate for slight excesses and deficiencies of most nutrients. (Compensation for excessive and deficient intakes of energy is less straightforward: see pp. 26–8 and 10–11, respectively.)

It is also possible to recognize sub-optimal states of nutrition, particularly with respect to deficiencies of vitamins, that are not sufficiently severe to classify as malnutrition. These marginal deficiency states are probably responsible for more ill-health in industrial societies than conditions of overt under-nutrition and deficiencies of several vitamins may occur together in the same individual. Marginal or sub-clinical nutritional deficiencies are by their very nature difficult to identify with any degree of certainty, since they do not present themselves in the form of well defined clinical signs or symptoms but they are real nevertheless. The symptoms are, in fact, quite non-specific and they vary with the individual and with the particular deficiency: tiredness, lassitude, depression, apathy, irritability and a general malaise are among the commonest ones observed and the same symptoms may occur in well nourished individuals for reasons quite unrelated to nutrition.

'Marginal nutritional excesses' do not constitute a problem since intakes of protein, vitamins and minerals two or three times physiological requirements do not result in any untoward effects. Intakes of quite small excesses of energy over and above requirements may, however, induce obesity in the long term.

1.2 Physiological requirements and recommended intakes (or allowances)

Every individual has a physiological requirement for each nutrient, i.e. the minimum amount of each which will maintain health in adults and permit normal growth in children. These requirements naturally vary according to age, sex and body weight but, in addition, there are considerable variations in requirements between individuals who in other respects are very similar. Thus, requirements should, ideally, be expressed in terms of a mean and standard deviation (SD) in order to quantify the extent of this variation. If, for example, the requirement of an adult man for a particular nutrient is expressed as 20 ± 2 mg day^{-1}, this means that 95% of all such men have a requirement within the range 16–24 mg day^{-1}, i.e. two SDs on either side of the mean and that 2.5% have a requirement below and 2.5% a requirement above this range (Fig. 1–1), assuming a normal distribution. Recommended daily intakes (RDIs) apply to populations and they are based on mean physiological requirements plus 2SDs plus appropriate 'safety margins'.

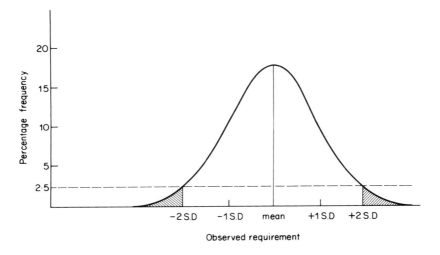

Fig. 1–1 Normal distribution curve for the observed (physiological) requirement for a particular nutrient. The minimum RDI (recommended daily intake) is the mean + 2 SD (standard deviation). The shaded 'tails' represent the 2.5% of the population with requirements lower or higher than the mean ± 2 SD. Thus, the minimum RDI should provide for the requirements of 97.5% of the population.

Many countries and the World Health Organization (WHO) and Food and Agriculture Organization (FAO) of the United Nations have published tables giving RDIs for all the most important nutrients for males and females according to age and in relation to pregnancy and lactation. RDIs are mainly used for planning purposes, e.g. in planning diets and food purchases for institutions such as schools, orphanages and mental hospitals and for expeditions, and for assessing the adequacy of the nutrient intake of populations whose food consumption has been estimated from dietary surveys, thus enabling groups with low intakes of particular nutrients to be identified. International agencies require to know how much food is needed for famine relief and for other programmes, and national governments need to calculate food supplies for their populations in relation to agricultural production and to food imports. In order to make the necessary calculations the average RDIs for the populations in question, based on their age and sex distribution, must be known.

A more recent use of RDIs, different in nature from the foregoing uses, is in relation to the 'nutritional labelling' of canned and packaged foods, which bear labels giving the proportion of the RDI of the most important nutrients provided by the contents of the pack or by a normal serving of it. Different criteria are used for establishing RDIs for the different nutrients and for energy.

Vitamins   The first step in determining RDIs for vitamins is to establish by experiment the minimum daily intake that will prevent the characteristic clinical signs and symptoms of deficiency from developing or cure these signs and symptoms once they have appeared. This often means that volunteers consume a diet grossly deficient in the vitamin under test, but adequate in all other respects, until signs of a deficiency appear. The minimum amount of the vitamin needed to cure the deficiency is then determined by giving graded doses of the pure vitamin. The resulting mean values ± SDs represent the starting points from which physiological requirements and RDIs evolve but it is clear from the previous discussion of conditions of marginal deficiency that the mere absence of clinical signs and symptoms is unlikely to indicate optimum nutrition. Additions have, therefore, to be made to these minima to provide a margin of safety against sub-clinical deficiencies and to ensure that the tissues have sufficient reserves of the vitamins to cover day to day fluctuations in intake and to provide for possible increases in requirement due to the stress and strains of everyday life. There is no general formula for deciding just how large these safety factors, different for different vitamins, should be, and traditionally it has been left to committees of experts to make recommendations on the basis of their combined wisdom and experience.

Recommendations for some of the less important vitamins, e.g. biotin and pantothenic acid, have not been determined with any degree of precision.

Minerals   The only minerals that figure in British tables of RDI are calcium and iron but magnesium, iodine and zinc are sometimes included in tables published in other countries. Requirements for calcium, phosphorus and magnesium are determined using the 'balance' techniques, i.e. by determining the minimum dietary supply that will ensure that losses from the body in urine and faeces equal the amount provided in the food. More balances have been carried out for calcium than for any other mineral because of the importance of this element in the normal growth and development of the skeleton and in various metabolic diseases of bone. Requirements for iron are based on the minimum amounts needed to maintain normal levels of haemoglobin in the blood and those for iodine on the amounts needed to prevent the development of goitre. In the case of iron, dietary requirements vary according to the nature of the diet: the iron present in plant materials is substantially less available than the iron of animal foods and the iron requirements of people consuming few or no foods of animal origin may be twice as high as those of people consuming a mixed diet.

As in the case of vitamins, in order to produce RDIs, additions have to be made to these minimum requirements to cater both for the needs of those with above average requirements and to provide a margin of safety.

Protein   The most satisfactory method for assessing protein requirements is by determining (by means of balance experiments) the lowest protein intake that will permit nitrogen equilibrium in adults and satisfactory growth and nitrogen retention in children. (On average, proteins contain 16% nitrogen and it is possible, therefore, to interconvert values for protein and nitrogen using this percentage.) A joint FAO/WHO *ad hoc* expert committee issued a report on Energy and Protein Requirements in 1973 in which the results of a number of such studies were collected together and the average nitrogen intake required to maintain balance in 75 subjects of both sexes, allowing a small amount of losses through the skin and for other minor losses, was 77 mg N per kg body weight per day when the dietary protein consisted of milk, egg, casein or a mixture of proteins including some of animal origin. The corresponding value when mixtures of plant protein were consumed was 93 mg N but when single sources of poor-quality plant proteins were consumed, a somewhat unrealistic situation except in the short term, the minimum requirement was up to 25% higher than this value.

Another method of estimating minimum requirements for protein is the 'factorial' method, whereby the minimum obligatory losses of nitrogen in the urine and faeces and through the skin when a nitrogen-free diet is consumed are totalled. For children this total is increased by the amount stored during growth, and for pregnant women by the amount stored in the foetus, foetal membranes and maternal tissue at the different stages of pregnancy. For lactating women, the amount of protein secreted in the milk must also be provided for.

When the minimum nitrogen requirements calculated by the factorial method are compared with the values obtained by the balance technique, the latter values are found to be about one-third higher than the former. This is not surprising, since it is known that dietary protein is not used with 100% efficiency by man: even when high quality proteins such as milk and eggs are given the efficiency with which their nitrogen is used is only about 70%. Thus, for example, an individual whose obligatory losses of nitrogen on a protein-free diet is 5 g would need approximately $5 \times 100/70 = 7.1$ g nitrogen, i.e. $7.1 \times 6.25 = 44$g protein of high quality per day to maintain nitrogen balance.

Table 1 summarizes the recommendations of the joint FAO/WHO expert committee and is reproduced by kind permission of the FAO. In the Table the calculated values for nitrogen requirements are averages and to derive RDIs or 'safe levels of intake' to use the expression favoured by the committee, these average values are increased by 30%, twice the coefficient of variation of 15% found in the nitrogen balance experiments, to ensure that the need of most of those individuals with the highest requirements are met. (The coefficient of variation is the standard deviation (SD) expressed as a percentage of the mean, i.e. (SD/mean) $\times$ 100.) It should be noted that these 'safe levels of intake' are for nitrogen in the form of a high quality protein such as milk or egg or a mixture of proteins equally high in quality. When proteins of inferior quality are consumed, larger amounts are needed to achieve nitrogen balance. The actual adjustment is based either on the protein score or on the net protein utilization (NPU) of the protein. Both these measures of protein quality derive numerical values for food proteins relative to egg or milk and the safe level of intake of any food protein is determined by the relationship:

$$\frac{\text{NPU (or chemical score) of egg or milk}}{\text{NPU of food protein}} \times \text{safe level of intake of egg or milk}$$

In 1975, the Committee on International Dietary Allowances of the International Union of Nutritional Sciences published a survey of recommended nutrient intakes in different countries. Protein allowances for young adult men varied from 53 to 85 g day^{-1} based on an NPU of 70. These differences reflect in

Table 1   Safe levels of intake of egg or milk protein.

Age	Total nitrogen requirements – obligatory losses and growth (mg nitrogen kg^{-1} day^{-1})		Adjusted nitrogen requirements – increased by 30% in accordance with balance and growth data (mg nitrogen kg^{-1} day^{-1})		Safe level of intake (adjusted requirement + 30% to allow for individual variability)			
					(mg nitrogen kg^{-1} day^{-1})		(g protein kg^{-1} day^{-1})	
(Months)								
<3					384a		2.40[a]	
3–5					296a		1.85[a]	
6–9	154		200		260		1.62	
9–11	136		177		230		1.44	
(Years)								
1	120		156		203		1.27	
2	112		146		190		1.19	
3	106		138		179		1.12	
4	100		130		169		1.06	
5	96		125		162		1.01	
6	92		120		156		0.98	
7	88		114		148		0.92	
8	83		108		140		0.87	
9	80		104		135		0.85	
	M	**F**	**M**	**F**	**M**	**F**	**M**	**F**
10	78	77	101	100	132	130	0.82	0.81
11	77	72	100	94	130	122	0.81	0.76
12	74	70	96	91	125	118	0.78	0.74
13	73	64	95	83	123	108	0.77	0.68
14	68	59	88	77	115	100	0.72	0.62
15	63	56	82	73	107	95	0.67	0.59
16	61	55	79	71	103	93	0.64	0.58
17	58	54	75	70	98	91	0.61	0.57
Adult	54	49	70	64	91	83	0.57	0.52

a   Based on observed intakes (mean + 2 standard deviations) of healthy infants. M, males;   F, females.

some measure the availability of foods in the different countries and, in general, recommendations are higher for affluent countries than for developing ones. In Britain, a report from the Department of Health and Social Security (DHSS) recommends a daily protein intake based on 10% of the energy intake and this gives an RDI for an adult man of 68 g. However, the DHSS report gives a *minimum* requirement of 45 g protein for men.

It is interesting to compare the safe level of protein intake recommended by the joint FAO/WHO committee, which is the lowest recommendation of any official body, with the intake of breast-fed infants, whose requirements are greater than at any other time of life. Breast milk contains 6–7% of its energy as protein and the 'safe level' of high quality protein recommended for adults by the FAO/WHO Committee works out to be 5–5.5% of the energy intake. This 'safe level' of protein intake is best regarded as equivalent to the upper limit of the normal range of physiological requirements and it is consistent with, i.e. somewhat less than, the 'natural intake' of breast-fed infants in relation to their energy intake. The RDIs of most countries are about twice physiological requirements to provide a margin of safety and to take account of the fact that the quality of the dietary protein is likely to be significantly less than that of egg or milk. Adjustments for protein quality are more important for children and pregnant and nursing women than for adult men and other women and there is some evidence that adult humans utilize essential amino acids more efficiently than rats when consuming sufficient protein to maintain nitrogen balance. It seems probable that some, perhaps all, of the essential amino acids are recycled to a greater extent in adult men and women than in the young growing rats that are used for NPU determinations and it may simply be that essential amino acids are used more efficiently for maintenance than for growth, rather than that there is a species difference between rats and men.

It must be emphasized that, in the words of the FAO/WHO committee on energy and protein requirements 'All estimates of protein requirements are valid only when energy requirements are fully met. When the total energy intake is inadequate, some dietary protein is used for energy and is not available to satisfy protein needs'.

Energy   Estimates of requirements for energy differ from those for other components of the diet in that no additions have to be made to provide a margin of safety and they are complicated by the fact that energy requirements vary according to climate, in particular to temperature, and to the physical activity of the individual and, therefore, of populations. A peasant population, engaged in hard manual work, clearly has a higher requirement for energy than a population of the same age and sex distribution engaged mainly in office work. Tables of energy requirements, therefore, take account of physical activity. Having said this, however, it must be stated that variations in energy requirements between individuals of the same age, sex, weight and physical activity are very great.

The extent of this variation is shown in Fig. 1–2 for adults and Fig. 1–3 for children. In both sexes some individuals of any particular age habitually consume twice as much energy per day as others and some one-year-old children eat more than some adults. Differences in basal metabolism, in physical activity

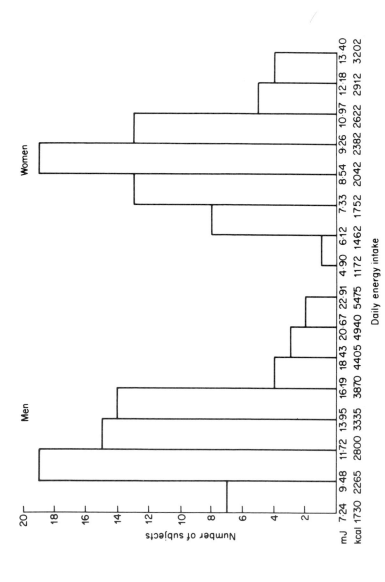

Fig. 1-2 Histogram showing the frequency distribution of daily energy intake of 63 men and 63 women (based on Fig. 1 of the paper 'Individual Variation' by E.M. Widdowson in Proceedings of the Nutrition Society, vol. 21 (1962) p. 122 and published by Cambridge University Press: reproduced by permission of the author and publisher).

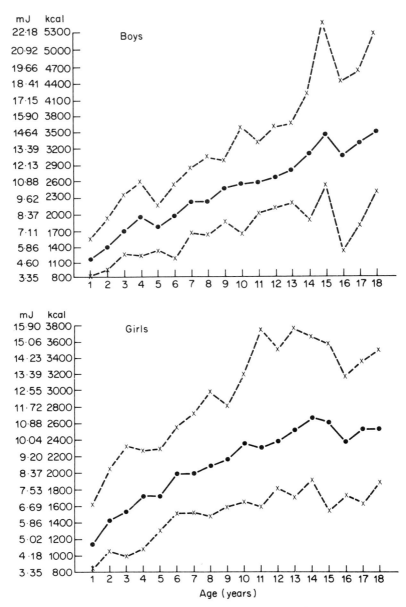

Fig. 1–3 Mean daily energy intake for boys and girls in relation to age (●): mean values for at least twenty at each age. Maximum and minimum intakes are also shown (X). (Values are taken from the Medical Research Council Special Report Series No.257 (1947) by E.M. Widdowson and published by permission of the Controller of Her Majesty's Stationery Office.)

and in the thermic effect of feeding (see pp. 26–7) are known to contribute to this variability and there may well be additional factors, but body weight is of minor importance.

Energy requirements may be assessed by measuring either food intake or energy expenditure and for individuals who are neither gaining nor losing weight the result should be the same by the two methods. The energy required by children is based on food consumption data. The extra energy required during pregnancy is calculated by the factorial method, i.e. by totalling the increase in basal metabolism (about 20% during the last trimester) and the energy stored in the foetus, foetal membranes and maternal tissue. The latest FAO/WHO committee recommended an average increase of 0.6 MJ day^{-1} in the first trimester and 1.5 MJ day^{-1} during the second and third trimesters. The additional energy required during lactation is related to the volume and energy content of the milk and to the efficiency of conversion of food energy into milk. For example, a woman secreting 800 ml milk day^{-1} would, assuming that the milk contains 2.9 MJ l^{-1} and that the efficiency of food energy conversion is 80%, requires to consume an additional $800/1000 \times 2.9 \times 100/80 = 2.9$ MJ day^{-1}.

Future developments Requirements and recommended intakes for many nutrients and for energy vary somewhat from country to country and the recommendations of any one authority are changed from time to time as new knowledge becomes available and as the results of older research are re-assessed. These processes of gradual change are bound to continue in the future but more radical changes should also be worked for. The first aim should be to establish well-founded tables of physiological requirements in the form of mean values ± SDs. These requirements would apply world wide, since there is no reason to believe that they vary between different ethnic groups, although appropriate correction factors for energy requirements in relation to temperature would have to be included as a footnote to the tables. Tables of physiological requirements for many of the major dietary components, including some of the essential amino acids, could be prepared now using existing information but reliable values for a number of vitamins and minerals have yet to be obtained. It should be noted that physiological requirements take account of the effects of the normal stress of everyday life but they do not provide for the additional requirements of sick or convalescing people.

The various national and international authorities would then use these physiological requirement values as a basis for preparing tables of RDIs for the populations they serve, taking account of the nature and amount of the foods normally available to them and of the margins of safety they consider appropriate to their conditions. Thus, far from being surprised at RDIs varying from country to country, one should expect this to happen.

2 Under-Nutrition and Related Conditions

2.1 Starvation, *anorexia nervosa* and protein-energy malnutrition

Starvation This is the most extreme form of under-nutrition: traditionally, one associates it with famine caused by natural disasters such as drought, floods or pestilence and with concentration camps, but starvation, partial or total, can also occur in circumstances nearer home, as for example in hunger strikes, in untreated coeliac disease (p. 41), *anorexia nervosa*, and *dysphagia* (in which patients have difficulty in swallowing).

Most healthy adults can lose 25% of their body weight as a result of starvation without suffering permanent damage. Table 2 shows the effect of this degree of starvation on body composition. Obese people can lose more than 25%, but danger to life increases progressively as loss of body weight increases beyond this limit.

Table 2 Changes in the body composition of an average man after losing 25% of his body weight due to starvation.

	Normal (kg)	After starvation (kg)	% loss
Protein	11.5	8.5	26
Fat	9.0	2.5	72
Carbohydrate	0.5	0.3	40
Water			
Extracellular	15.0	15.0	0
Intracellular	25.0	19.0	24
Minerals	4.0	3.5	12
Total body weight	65	48.8	25

Tissue wasting and weight loss are rapid in the initial stages of starvation but the rate of loss gradually slows down as adaptive changes, evolved presumably in response to early man's exposure to intermittent food supplies, come into play. In the first few days of starvation, 1.5–2 kg of weight may be lost, due mainly to losses of glycogen, protein and water and the same phenomenon is observed in the early stages of dieting (p. 29). During the first week of starvation, nitrogen excretion in the urine falls from perhaps 12 g d^{-1} (equivalent to 75 g protein) to 6 g d^{-1} after 3 d, reaching a minimum of about 4.7 g d^{-1} after several weeks of starvation. The adaptive changes serve to conserve body protein, to provide the minimum glucose for essential metabolic purposes (e.g. for the red cells and the brain) and to utilize fat stores to the maximum extent. The brain normally uses glucose as an energy source but in starvation ketone bodies (derived from fat) replace glucose to an increasing extent.

It is not possible to adapt fully to complete starvation but adaptation to semi-starvation can be virtually complete. In the well-known 'Minnesota experiment' 32 men spent six weeks on mean energy intakes less than half of normal (6.57 compared with 14.62 MJ d^{-1}) and at the end of this time they had almost regained energy balance at their new reduced body weight by reducing basal metabolism and physical activity: the thermic effect of feeding (pp. 26–7) was also lower.

Prolonged starvation is characterized by extreme muscle wasting, a loose dry skin, oedema and low pulse rate and blood pressure. Severe personality changes may occur and the mind becomes wholly obsessed with thoughts of food. The rehabilitation of starving people is not difficult provided that atrophy of, and degenerative changes in, the organs and systems of the body have not progressed too far: all they need is food. In cases of extreme and prolonged starvation, however, rehabilitation can be hazardous and even fatal unless extreme care is exercised. In this condition, the smooth muscles, the glands and the mucosa (the layer of absorptive cells) of the intestines atrophy and the walls become almost paper-thin. If the powers of digestion and absorption are completely lost, death is inevitable, but if some digestive function remains there is hope of recovery. Bland, highly digestible foods should be given in very small meals, particularly if there is diarrhoea. Cooked baby cereal made up with skimmed milk and given in the form of a thin porridge is ideal but not always available. Once the victim is taking food well, increasing amounts should be given to satisfy the appetite.

Anorexia nervosa   This is a disease of psychiatric origin in which the patient refuses to eat. It can be fatal. It occurs most frequently in adolescent girls and young women between the ages of 15 and 25 but it can also occur in older women and in men. Once a very rare condition, its prevalence seems to have increased in recent years, mainly among the middle-classes. Its essential feature is an obsessional wish to avoid any suspicion of plumpness and it has been called the 'slimmer's disease', because it often develops from a normal desire to slim by dieting. Patients exhibit a completely distorted view of their bodily conformation: whereas they are, in fact, extremely thin and emaciated, they insist that they are fat. It is as though they are permanently looking at themselves in a distorting mirror located in their mind's eye. The medical and psychological histories of patients show few common features but many are anxious and insecure, possibly as a result of family conflicts. They are depressed, and many have psycho-sexual problems. In true anorexia the patients lose all desire to eat and in the initial stages of their rehabilitation intravenous feeding may have to be resorted to. There is another psychiatric condition, similar in some respects to anorexia, in which patients have continually to repress the desire to eat. Sometimes, they give way to this desire and engage in huge binges, after which they may deliberately vomit the contents of their stomachs or purge themselves repeatedly.

In treating anorexia nervosa, the basic problem, of course, is to get the patient to eat. Since anorexia nervosa is a psychiatric disease, successful treatment must include a psychiatric component. If the condition is not to recur once normal weight has been regained as a result of hospital treatment, the patient needs continuous support and understanding from family and friends and the help of the psychiatric social worker.

Protein energy-malnutrition   In a global context, protein-energy malnutrition (PEM) in children in third-world countries is the most serious nutritional disease of all, both quantitatively, in terms of the vast numbers involved, and qualitatively, in terms of the human misery it encompasses. In some under-developed countries, one-third of all children born die before reaching the age of five either from PEM itself or from the diseases that accompany it. The term PEM covers a wide spectrum of clinical conditions: the two extremes are *marasmus* and *kwashiorkor* and there are various intermediate conditions between these extremes. Before discussing the detailed clinical features of these conditions, a brief consideration of normal growth in children is appropriate.

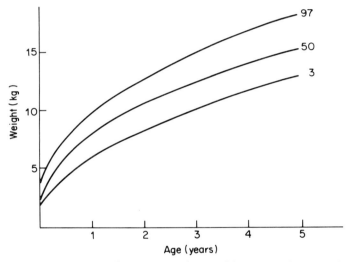

Fig. 2–1 Standard growth chart for boys up to the age of 5 years showing curves for the 3rd, 50th and 97th centiles. (Height charts are similar.)

Although individual children vary greatly in their rate of growth, in terms of both height and weight, standard growth charts for both sexes have been prepared by different research groups relating age to height and weight (Fig. 2–1). A number of standard growth lines are drawn on these charts representing 'high', 'low' and 'medium' rates of growth. The last, the so-called 50th percentile line represents the median growth line, while the 3rd and 97th percentiles represent the lines for the 3% of the population with, respectively, the lowest and highest rates of growth. The growth curve of a normal child runs parallel to the percentile lines but when growth falters and the curve falls below the percentile line on which it started this constitutes a danger signal that PEM is imminent.

Kwashiorkor occurs mainly in older infants and young children who have been under-nourished with respect to energy and protein for some time. These children are apathetic but the most characteristic feature of the condition is oedema, in which fluid accumulates under the skin, particularly of the face (giving the characteristic 'moon' face), hands and feet. Other features include an enlarged liver, infiltrated with fat, a serious reduction of the plasma albumin level, a distorted serum amino acid pattern and a characteristic flaking of the skin and depigmentation of the hair. The muscles are severely wasted but this is obscured by the oedema. The disease is often precipitated by an attack of measles, malaria, gastro-enteritis or some other condition that induces anorexia.

Marasmus is most common in infants. It is characterized by gross wasting of muscles, extreme emaciation and a loose skin but the liver is not enlarged nor is oedema present. In this type of PEM infants are more often irritable than apathetic and their appetite is usually good.

Why do some under-nourished children develop kwashiorkor while others become marasmic? The classical explanation is that kwashiorkor is induced by a chronic deficiency of protein associated with an adequate intake of energy, whereas marasmus results when intakes of both protein and energy are deficient for prolonged periods. This explanation will most probably need to be modified in the future as there is a good deal of evidence that intake of energy is also inadequate in kwashiorkor and the precise combination of circumstances (in terms of dietary intakes of energy and protein) that precipitates the two extreme manifestations of PEM is not fully understood, nor is it known why so many children develop the intermediate form of PEM (marasmic kwashiorkor) which is more common than either of the two ends of the PEM spectrum. It is possible, however, to identify a number of unfavourable conditions that are associated with one form or other of PEM, namely early weaning from the breast; bulky weaning and pre-weaning foods low in both energy and protein; dilute milk formulae prepared unhygienically; infectious diseases, including intestinal parasites; poverty and ignorance; broken homes.

The hormonal status in marasmus and that in kwashiorkor are somewhat different: in particular, the circulating level of cortisol is higher in the former condition. It has been suggested that the endocrine system of the marasmic child has adapted to the protein-energy deficiency whereas that of the child suffering from kwashiorkor has failed to adapt. Kwashiorkor is certainly the more serious of the two conditions in terms of survival rate. In marasmus, the amino acid pattern of the plasma is less seriously distorted due to the more effective mobilization of muscle protein to maintain the essential functions of the liver. In the present context, the formation of plasma albumin and the synthesis of the apoprotein needed to transport the lipids from the liver in the form of lipoproteins are the most important of these functions.

The central argument of the 'failure to adapt' hypothesis of kwashiorkor may be summarized as follows. In the development of marasmus the blood sugar and insulin levels fall in response to the low energy intake, and the blood sugar is maintained at this lower level by increased secretion of cortisol, the main action of which is to mobilize amino acids from muscle protein. Some of these amino acids are used by the liver for the synthesis of the vital proteins noted above, while others are deaminated and the residues converted into glucose for the maintenance of the blood sugar level. In kwashiorkor, the energy intake, in particular the carbohydrate intake, is sufficiently high to maintain higher levels of blood sugar and insulin than in marasmus, with the result that the stimulus to cortisol secretion is less. The body is not then able to supplement the small amounts of amino acids coming from the food with sufficient amino acids from the muscle to enable the liver to maintain normal functions.

Children suffering from PEM are often anaemic and deficiencies of nutrients such as vitamin A, nicotinic acid and other vitamins of the B group, trace minerals and essential fatty acids often accompany PEM.

There is a widely-held view that malnutrition in infancy and childhood may produce permanent, irreversible damage to the brain sufficiently great to impair intellectual development and to cause serious mental retardation. The evidence to support this thesis is not particularly strong but it is a possibility that must be recognized and taken seriously. A major practical difficulty in testing this theory is that most malnourished children suffer multiple deprivation so that it is not possible to separate their nutritional from their social and psychological environments and there can be no doubt that a child's ultimate intellectual status (in terms of IQ) is the end product of a complex interaction between all these environmental factors and his genetic make-up.

In adults PEM occurs as a result of partial or total starvation. It usually takes the form of marasmus but the condition known as famine oedema is the adult equivalent of kwashiorkor. In recent years a disturbingly high incidence of PEM has been reported in patients about to undergo surgical operations, particularly for cancer and for diseases of the gastro-intestinal tract. The chance of any particular operation being successful is substantially less and post-operative complications are significantly more common and more serious in a malnourished than in a well-fed patient. Many surgeons are now assessing the nutritional status of their patients before surgery by arm circumference and skinfold thickness measurements or by hand-grip strength tests and any that are found to be seriously malnourished are given special feeding to restore their wasted tissues before the operation.

2.2   Vitamin and mineral deficiencies

Anaemias   Anaemia is a condition in which there is a reduced concentration of haemoglobin (Hb) in the blood. The normal range of Hb concentrations in men is 13–17 g 100 ml^{-1} and in women 12–16 g 100 ml^{-1} (with the lower point on the range reduced to 11 g 100 ml^{-1} during pregnancy when the blood volume increases considerably) and Hb concentrations below these ranges indicate anaemia. Anaemia may be caused by excessive blood loss, e.g. by hook-worm infection in tropical countries, by an abnormally high rate of red cell destruction (e.g. in sickle-cell anaemia) or by nutritional deficiencies. Emphasis will be placed here on the nutritional, causes.

The most important nutrients, a deficiency of which results in anaemia, are iron, folic acid and vitamin B_{12}, but anaemia also occurs in copper, pyridoxine and vitamin E deficiency and in PEM. A mild anaemia may not produce any symptoms at all in people in sedentary occupations but any unaccustomed activity, such as running upstairs, or any sustained physical activity causes breathlessness. A severe anaemia seriously impairs the ability to carry out hard physical work.

Iron deficiency anaemia is one of the most prevalent diseases of nutritional origin throughout the world. It affects mainly women of child-bearing age but it may also occur in infants and young children. In many developing countries a primary nutritional deficiency of iron is a serious public health problem and Hb concentrations as low as 5 g 100 ml^{-1} or even less are not uncommon. Even in prosperous countries the incidence of some degree of this type of anaemia is 10–15% in young and middle-aged women. In these populations, a primary nutritional deficiency is not the cause of this condition; rather, it is the result of heavy blood loss during menstruation. The only way in which iron can be lost from the body in significant amounts is by bleeding. It is not possible to provide for the high iron requirements of women who lose abnormally large amounts of blood during menstruation and supplementary iron must be given in the form of tablets. Requirements for iron are increased during pregnancy when, once again, supplementation of the diet is desirable.

Iron is absorbed mainly in the upper part of the small intestine but some absorption also occurs in the stomach and the ileum. The absorption of iron from a mixed western-type diet is very low, ranging from a mean of 6% in normal men to 14% in women. More iron is absorbed in an iron-deficiency than when the iron status of the body is high and less is absorbed when the secretion of hydrochloric acid into the stomach is impaired. The iron present in cereals and other plant products is mainly in the form of inorganic iron and only 1–5% of this iron is absorbed. Soya beans are exceptional in that the iron present is more readily available and it may be absorbed to the extent of 7–8%. Reducing compounds, in particular, ascorbic acid (vitamin C), increase the extent to which inorganic iron is absorbed, probably by increasing the proportion present in the Fe^{2+} (ferrous) state.

Most of the iron present in muscle (meat) and in other animal tissues is present in organic combination as the haem molecule and iron in this form is much more efficiently absorbed than inorganic iron. Absorption of haem iron is not influenced by reducing compounds and the iron in meat is absorbed to the extent of 10–20%. Eggs are relatively rich in iron but it is poorly absorbed because of the phosphoproteins present in the yolk. Other phosphorus-containing compounds, notably the phytates present in the outer layers of cereal grains, also interfere with the absorption of iron.

Prolonged iron deficiency causes a number of abnormal conditions in addition to anaemia – dry and brittle hair and finger nails, a smooth moist tongue, due to loss of papillae, and difficulty in swallowing, due to the development of a mucosal web in the upper part of the oesophagus.

The mean obligatory daily loss of iron in men and post-menopausal women is about 1 mg and in younger women at least double this amount. The maximum percentage of iron that can be absorbed from a mixed diet is about 20% and since the mean daily intake may be only 10 mg (the mean intake in Britain is about 12 mg d^{-1}) it is not difficult to see why women with an above-average requirement for iron are liable to become anaemic In some under-developed countries, the mean daily intake of iron may be as little as 6 mg.

Iron-deficiency anaemia is common in infants in many parts of the world but it no longer occurs to any significant extent in western countries except perhaps in pre-term infants. At birth the full-term baby has a very high Hb level, about 17 g 100 ml^{-1} blood. During the first few weeks after birth, the older red cells containing foetal Hb are broken down and the Hb settles down at a concentration of 11–12 g 100 ml^{-1}. The iron released from the worn out cells is stored, mainly in the liver. The milk of all species of mammal is naturally very low in iron (1–2 mg l^{-1}), far too little to supply the requirements of the infant but the amount of iron stored in the liver during intra-uterine development and during the first few weeks after birth are sufficient to last for at least four months even if the infant is fed on nothing but breast milk. Infants of low birth weight and those born to iron-deficient mothers are likely to have much smaller stores of iron than normal and these babies are likely to benefit from the iron added to commercial infant milks.

Folic acid is the generic term for a complex group of naturally occurring compounds derived from pteroylmonoglutamic acid and containing a variable number of molecules of glutamic acid, up to a total of seven. These compounds are most abundant in green leafy vegetables, mushrooms, pulses, white fish, liver and yeast but most fruits and cereals are, at best, only fair dietary source. Milk, perhaps surprisingly, is a poor source and goat's milk is particularly deficient. Uncertainties about the amount and precise nature of the folate compounds in foods and the extent to which these various compounds are absorbed make it virtually impossible to know just how much folate is available from any particular food. Furthermore, cooking can cause substantial losses of folic acid.

A deficiency of this vitamin causes a megaloblastic anaemia in which the red cells are pale and enlarged and the bone marrow shows characteristic changes. In folate deficiency DNA synthesis is impaired and since bone marrow is the tissue in which cell division (associated with the production of both red and white blood cells), proceeds most rapidly, it is this tissue that is first to show signs of a folate deficiency. The anaemia that results from this deficiency is due partly to a reduced rate of production of new red cells and partly to a decreased life-span of the red cells from a normal life of 120 d to 20–70 d. The cells of the intestinal villi also divide rapidly and these cells, too, suffer degenerative changes in a folic acid deficiency.

A folic acid deficiency can be caused either by consuming a diet deficient in the vitamin, as in many poor countries in tropical regions of the world, or by a failure to absorb the vitamin, as in various malabsorption syndromes. If these circumstances coincide with a period when requirements for folic acid are increased, as during pregnancy or during periods of rapid growth, the seriousness of the resulting anaemia will be increased. Even in prosperous countries, megaloblastic anaemia is not uncommon in pregnancy, particularly with multiple birth pregnancies. Marrow changes occur in 25–30% of all women during pregnancy, and supplementary folic acid is often prescribed for pregnant women during the last trimester. There are seasonal differences in the megaloblastic anaemia of pregnancy. In Britain, the highest incidence is in the winter and early spring when consumption of fresh vegetables, particularly lettuce, is low. Folic acid deficiency sometimes affects premature infants if they are born with low reserves, especially when they are growing rapidly.

Vitamin B_{12} deficiency   Addisonian pernicious anaemia is one of the classical anaemias. Until 1926, when the beneficial effect of raw liver in causing a remission of the disease was demonstrated, it was invariably fatal. It is now known to be due to a deficiency of vitamin B_{12} brought about by a failure to absorb the vitamin. Whereas raw minced beef will not cure the disease, raw beef that has spent a few hours in the stomach of a healthy person will. The explanation of this extraordinary fact is that normal gastric juice contains a specific glycoprotein, the so-called intrinsic factor, essential for the absorption of vitamin B_{12}, and this protein is absent in patients suffering from pernicious anaemia. Normal gastric juice by itself is ineffective, as it does not contain the vitamin. In pernicious anaemia the gastric glands that produce the intrinsic factor are destroyed by an auto-immune reaction and the disease, in fact, should be regarded as an auto-immune disease in which the body produces antibodies directed against its own proteins.

The anaemia resulting from a deficiency of vitamin B_{12} is haematologically indistinguishable from that occurring in a folic acid deficiency and the metabolism of the two vitamins is closely interrelated. In a vitamin B_{12} deficiency, there is a shortage of the active form of folate required in DNA biosynthesis and pernicious anaemia does in fact respond to treatment with folic acid. However, no megaloblastic anaemia should be treated with folic acid unless and until the possibility of a vitamin B_{12} deficiency has been completely eliminated.

Vitamin B_{12} is found naturally only in foods of animal origin and in some products of fermentation. Virtually all the molecules of vitamin B_{12} found in the world today originate in microbial cells and most of the vitamin B_{12} present in human tissues originated in the bacteria that inhabit the fore-stomachs of ruminant animals. These bacteria are killed in the true stomach and the vitamin B_{12} liberated after the cells are digested is transported along the digestive tract in combination with the intrinsic factor, and absorbed in the lower ileum. The vitamin is then stored in the tissues or secreted in the milk.

Plant foods do not contain any vitamin B_{12}, except in so far as they are contaminated by micro-organisms, and strict vegetarians (vegans) who do not consume animal products, even eggs, milk or cheese, are liable to develop a primary nutritional deficiency of the vitamin unless fermented plant products form a regular part of their diet. It is something of a mystery why vitamin B_{12} deficiency is not more common in vegans than it actually is and experts are still arguing as to whether or not the micro-organisms inhabiting the lower bowel supply any vitamins of the B group to their host. Experiments with laboratory animals suggest that the only way in which the vitamins synthesized by the intestinal bacteria can be made available to the host animal is by coprophagy, i.e. by ingestion of the faeces.

Anaemia is not the only feature of a vitamin B_{12} deficiency: there are also serious neurological complications, involving both the peripheral nerves and the central nervous system, and whereas the anaemia is readily cured, the nervous lesions are incurable when they reach an advanced stage.

In some countries raw fish is considered to be a delicacy and as a result of this practice infestation of the population with a particular species of fish tape-worm is not uncommon (2% of the adult population in Finland). These worms absorb vitamin B_{12} from the intestinal contents, thus inducing a deficiency of the vitamin that may lead to anaemia. Bacterial infections of the small intestine can have a similar effect.

Rickets and osteomalacia   Rickets is a disease of children characterized by a failure of the growing bones to calcify normally. In infants and young children the most striking features of rickets are bow-legs and 'beading' (enlargement) of the junctions of the ribs on the side of the chest but in older children and adolescents knock-knees are more characteristic of the disease. Other bones of the skeleton are seriously deformed in severe cases and deformities of the pelvic girdle in females may lead to difficulties in child-birth many years later.

Osteomalacia is the corresponding disease in adults. It is most common in women of child-bearing age, particularly after repeated pregnancies. Bone tissue undergoes a continuous process of destruction and formation throughout life and in osteomalacia the newly-formed bone is poorly calcified and the skeleton is less able to perform its supportive function. Osteomalacia is usually associated with severe skeletal pain, particularly in the lower back, but the legs, ribs and other sites may also be affected and show tenderness when subjected to pressure.

These diseases are caused by a deficiency of vitamin D and they may be exacerbated by a simultaneous deficiency of calcium. The distribution of vitamin D in foods is somewhat limited: the best natural sources are oily fish, fortified margarine, liver and eggs. Butter, cheese and unfortified milk are, at best, only fair sources, and meat, cereals and indeed all plant foods, are devoid of the vitamin.

Vitamin D is the only vitamin, apart from nicotinic acid, that is synthesized in the body. Vitamin D is produced in the skin on exposure to sunlight or to artificial sources of ultra-violet (u.v.) light. The anti-rachitic potency of sunlight, i.e. its ability to convert the precursor of vitamin D in the skin to the active vitamin, is greater in summer than in winter and greater at low than at high latitudes. The 'natural' form of the vitamin thus generated is called D_3 and the form used to fortify foods is known as D_2: the latter is produced by irradiating the plant sterol, ergosterol.

Rickets occurs wherever infants and young children are kept indoors, even in tropical countries, if the milk, cereals and other foods they are given are not fortified with vitamin D, unless they are given supplementary vitamin D in the form of fish-liver oil or some other pharmaceutical preparation. In Britain, rickets appeared to have been conquered by the end of the second world war but it became a major public health problem from the early 1960s, when it reappeared in Glasgow and in the large industrial cities of Scotland and the north of England among the children of Asian immigrants. Why are Asians in Britain so much more susceptible to rickets (and osteomalacia, as we now know) than West Indians, for example, or the indigenous white population? The answer to this question is still not certain but it seems probable that a number of factors are involved. Earlier theories that sought to implicate the chappati (which was thought to induce a deficiency of calcium by virtue of its high phytate content) or suggested that people with pigmented skins are less efficient at utilizing the u.v. rays of the sun for vitamin D synthesis (because a high proportion of the u.v radiation is absorbed by the melanin pigment) are almost certainly incorrect. A low dietary intake of vitamin D may provide a partial answer to the question but it seems probable that a major factor is that Asian children play outside less than other children and they wear more clothes so that a smaller area of their skin is exposed to the sun's rays. This is particularly true for adolescents. The fact that the incidence of Asian rickets is higher in girls, who for reasons of culture, tradition and religion spend less time outside the home than boys, is consistent with this theory. One reason for the greater incidence of rickets in Glasgow and Bradford than in London may be the higher u.v potency of sunlight in the south than in the north of Britain In recent years, there have been radical changes in thinking about the importance of the diet in providing for the body's requirements for vitamin D; whereas it used to be thought that the diet provided the major source of the vitamin, it is now certain that the diet is a minor source for all people except for those who are house-bound and for those who consume unusually large amounts of vitamin D-rich foods. Despite the fact that most people obtain the major proportion of their vitamin D by exposing their skin to sunlight, it is important for children and adults who, for any reason, do not spend sufficient time out of doors to generate adequate amounts of the vitamin, to be given supplementary vitamin D.

Vitamin D is very toxic when taken in excess and care must be exercized when supplementary vitamin D is used. Infants are particularly susceptible to vitamin D intoxication. Fortunately, there is no danger of poisoning by excessive exposure to the sun: even in the life guards who patrol sub-tropical holiday beaches the plasma concentrations of the circulating form of vitamin D is far below that observed in people intoxicated with the vitamin.

Ascorbic acid (Vitamin C) deficiency The classical disease associated with a deficiency of vitamin C is scurvy, the scourge of seafarers in the days of sail. It is recorded that, during Vasco de Gama's famous voyage to India round the Cape of Good Hope in 1497, 100 of his crew of 160 died of this disease. At the present time, a deficiency of ascorbic acid is relatively uncommon but it sometimes occurs in old people living alone, particularly widowers, who are unable to look after themselves properly.

Man and his near relations in the animal kingdom are almost unique among warm-blooded animals in requiring a dietary source of vitamin C. Apart from primates, the only animals that are unable to synthesize the vitamin in their own tissues are guinea pigs and some fruit-eating birds and bats. The best natural sources of ascorbic acid are fresh fruit and vegetables but there are considerable variations between species in their content of the vitamin: citrus fruits, strawberries and green peppers are excellent sources and blackcurrants contain even more of the vitamin: tomatoes, lettuces and all green leafy vegetables are also good sources when eaten raw. Among foods of animal origin, liver is the best source. Considerable losses occur during cooking due to irreversible oxidation but these losses can be minimized by cooking for as short a time as possible, by avoiding delays in serving once the food has been cooked and by not using either copper saucepans or bicarbonate of soda when cooking vegetables. Losses also occur between the time that leafy vegetables are cut and eaten, due to the wilting process.

Ascorbic acid is essential for the normal metabolism of connective tissue, in particular, for the biosynthesis of collagen and the intercellular matrix or ground substance. The most characteristic features of scurvy are associated with capillary haemorrhages, due to a weakening of the walls of the capillaries. The gums become red and swollen and bleed easily and often become secondarily infected: pin-point haemorrhages occur around the hair follicles and patients bruise easily and often show subcutaneous haemorrhages on the feet and ankles. Wounds and fractures fail to heal – both processes are dependent on collagen synthesis – and osteoporosis often accompanies scurvy in the elderly. Clinical signs of scurvy occur only when the deficiency of vitamin C is severe: in a mild deficiency, mental symptoms, depression and hysteria, are the first to appear; fatigue and lassitude are also early signs of sub-clinical deficiency of the vitamin.

In the late nineteenth century, scurvy was not uncommon in infants fed on condensed or evaporated milk. At the present time these milks are labelled 'not fit for infants' but in spite of this warning infantile scurvy occasionally occurs in babies fed on tinned milk.

The most reliable biochemical test of ascorbic acid status is the amount present in the leucocytes: plasma levels provide a less reliable indicator of tissue stores. Surveys have shown that the mean concentration of ascorbic acid in the leucocytes is higher in women than in men and lower in smokers than in non-smokers. At one time it was thought that smoking somehow affected the metabolism of vitamin C but a more probable explanation is that smokers have different dietary habits from non-smokers, i.e. their consumption of vitamin C-rich foods is less, possibly because they have lost their sense of taste and with it their ability to appreciate the subtle flavours of fresh, natural foods.

Drug-induced vitamin deficiencies   Many drugs exert their action by influencing the activity of particular enzymes and by changing the rate or direction of a particular metabolic reaction and since all the vitamins of the B group act as co-factors in enzymic reactions it is not to be wondered at that drugs and vitamins interact in some instances to produce unexpected and undesirable side-effects. Some of the best known of these interactions are mentioned below and, with the introduction of new drugs, it is likely that further examples will appear in the future.

Folic acid antagonists are used in cancer chemotherapy. They act by interfering with the biosynthesis of DNA in tumour cells but they also affect normal cells in the same way. Fortunately, the tumour cells are more susceptible to the drugs than normal cells and alternate treatment with drug and with folate usually prevents the development of a folate deficiency. Some anti-convulsant drugs used in the long-term treatment of epileptics, e.g. phenobarbital and diphenylhydantoin, induce a megaloblastic anaemia responsive to folate but how these drugs interfere with the metabolism of folic acid is not known.

The drug isoniazid, widely used in the treatment of tuberculosis, combines with pyridoxal phosphate, the active co-enzyme form of vitamin B_6, thereby inducing a deficiency of the vitamin and it is standard practice to administer large doses of vitamin B_6 together with isoniazid. A secondary action of this drug is to cause pellagra, a disease due to nicotinic acid deficiency This vitamin is synthesized in the body from the essential amino acid tryptophan by a long and devious pathway that involves vitamin B_6-dependent enzymes at several stages. Thus, isoniazid induces a secondary deficiency of vitamin B_6 which in turn induces a tertiary deficiency of nicotinic acid.

Oral contraceptive drugs can cause a mild vitamin B_6-deficiency associated with psychological depression by speeding-up the flow of tryptophan through the nicotinic acid pathway, thus increasing the requirement for vitamin B_6. The depression is thought to be due to a slight deficiency in the production of the neurotransmitter serotonin, the precursor of which is tryptophan. Biosynthesis of this transmitter is also vitamin B_6 dependent, so the contraceptive steroids reduce the amount of both its starting material and its co-factor. This effect is due to the oestrogenic component of the oral contraceptive pill and the danger is reduced by lowering the oestrogen content of the pill. High circulating levels of oestrogen occur naturally during pregnancy and a slight deficiency of vitamin B_6 sometimes occurs at this time.

Alcoholism   Alcoholic drinks form very incomplete diets, and alcoholics, who obtain a substantial proportion of their total energy requirements from these beverages, are likely, therefore, to suffer from deficiencies of a number of different nutrients. The vitamin deficiencies most commonly involved are thiamin, folic acid, nicotinic acid and vitamin B_6. Alcoholics may also be deficient in potassium, magnesium and zinc and multiple deficiencies of vitamins, minerals and protein may be combined in one individual. A good mixed diet is, therefore, an essential prerequisite for the rehabilitation of alcoholics.

However, these deficiency conditions are not usually responsible for these people finding themselves in hospital. If they do not have a car accident or end up in a special psychiatric unit, cirrhosis of the liver is the usual reason for entering hospital, although carcinoma of the oesophagus and stomach, pancreatitis, gastritis and chronic heart failure are other diseases that are more frequent in alcoholics than in non-alcoholics. Even more serious than the physical consequences of alcoholism, however, is the psychological deterioration of the individual, that is a feature of all drug addiction, and the consequent breakdown of family and social relationships.

Vitamin A deficiency   is not a problem in affluent societies in which milk and dairy products, eggs and fortified margarine, all valuable sources of the vitamin, are common items of diet. In a global context, however, it is the most serious primary nutritional deficiency after PEM and it is one of the major causes of blindness in tropical countries. A vitamin A deficiency often accompanies PEM in children, due either to a primary nutritional deficiency of the vitamin or to a deficiency of the specific protein that transports the vitamin in the plasma, the so-called retinol-binding protein. Of the staple cereals, yellow maize is the only one with significant vitamin A potency, so that populations subsisting on rice, wheat and sorghum are at risk of a deficiency. Among the starchy roots that form the staple diet of many people in the wet tropics, the sweet potato is the only one that provides a reasonable source of the carotenoid pigments that act as precursors of vitamin A. Vitamin A itself is found only in animal products and the carotenoid pigments, on average, are only about one-sixth as potent weight for weight as vitamin A itself, partly because they are less well absorbed than the active vitamin and partly because the efficiency with which they are converted is rather low, 50% or less.

In order to avoid a deficiency of vitamin A, populations that subsist on a staple diet deficient in the vitamin, e.g. rice or cassava, must supplement their diet with dairy products or with carotene-containing fruits and vegetables. All green leafy vegetables and yellow or orange coloured fruits and vegetables, such as melons, apricots, yellow peaches, pumpkins, tomatoes and carrots, contain useful amounts of carotene pigments. Red palm oil, used extensively for cooking in West Africa, is a very rich source of pro-vitamin A.

Changing the dietary habits of a population takes a long time, even where economic constraints are not limiting, and in countries where keratomalacia, the type of blindness caused by a deficiency of vitamin A, is a serious problem, short-term emergency measures must be taken. Although vitamin A is toxic when taken in excessive amounts, large single doses of the order of 50 mg given every six months are very effective in preventing vitamin A deficiency in children. Pregnant and nursing women are also at risk and they too should be given supplementary vitamin A. Fortification of a staple food as a preventive measure has also been successful in a number of countries. In Guatemala sugar (sucrose) has been used as the vehicle for fortification and in the Philippines mono-sodium glutamate, universally used for flavouring stews, has been tried. Wherever feasible, food fortification is the method of choice, as the whole population is treated. Furthermore, it is much cheaper than individual dosing. There are, however, many practical problems to be overcome before any food fortification programme can be successfully mounted.

Other primary vitamin deficiencies   Most vitamin deficiencies occur in people consuming diets consisting mainly of one staple food or of a restricted number of foods all of which are deficient in the same vitamin or vitamins. Few people consume a restricted diet from choice, and poverty always has been, and probably always will be, the major cause of under-nutrition. There are, however, certain food cults, the members of which consume very peculiar diets. Many unusual diets are perfectly adequate for maintaining health but some are responsible for inducing serious nutritional deficiencies. The Zen Macrobiotic diet in its most extreme form (Diet 7) is extremely dangerous and has caused many deaths and much needless suffering. This diet consists wholly of cereals, in particular, of brown rice, and strict adherents to this diet soon develop scurvy, anaemia, and other vitamin deficiencies. In infants and young children subjected to this and similar diets PEM is an additional danger.

Beri-beri, the classical deficiency disease of rice-eating populations of the Far East is now much less common than in earlier years due to a combination of circumstances, including a general improvement and diversification of the diet, the use of less highly milled rice, the technique of par-boiling before milling, whereby some of the thiamin is leached out from the bran and absorbed by the grain, and fortification of rice with thiamin. However, the disease still occurs in rural populations in which these desirable dietary changes have not taken place.

Pellagra, the disease of maize- and sorghum-eating peoples, is also less common than in the past but it still constitutes a serious problem in parts of India and Africa. Whereas it used to be common among the poor farmers and farm and mill workers in the southern states of the USA up to 1940, it is now quite rare in that country. Pellagra was recognized as a condition of nicotinic acid deficiency in 1937 but this recognition was not the reason for the virtual disappearance of the disease a few years after the link between pellagra and nicotinic acid was discovered. This disappearance was in fact due to an increase in the purchasing power of the people of the region associated with the industrial development which followed the outbreak of the Second World War. People only subsist on a diet of maize if they cannot afford anything better and as soon as their economic condition improves they immediately start to eat a more varied diet as a first call on their increased income.

Maize (Indian Corn) is native to the Americas and it is interesting to enquire why the Indians of North and South America did not develop pellagra in pre-colonial times. The probable explanation is that their diet was not restricted entirely to maize, but the method of preparing the grain may also have been a factor. Some of the tribes in North America roast the corn on the cob over a fire and this treatment liberates the nicotinic acid from the unavailable complex in which it is present in the grain. In Mexico, the maize meal is soaked in lime-water overnight before it is cooked and this treatment, too, renders the nicotinic acid available.

Other mineral deficiencies   After iron, the most widespread mineral deficiency condition occurring in man is that of iodine. It is caused by a deficiency of the element in the soil and there are iodine-deficient areas in all continents. Crops grown on mineral-deficient soils are themselves deficient in the same minerals so that human populations that subsist largely or wholly on locally-produced foods become deficient in the elements in which the soil is lacking. In developed countries with good transport, there is much inter-change of foods between different regions and from abroad and the risk of any particular mineral deficiency occurring is thereby reduced. A serious deficiency of iodine occurs, therefore, mainly in populations living off the land in remote and isolated regions, although a mild deficiency of the element occurs in a small proportion of individuals in many, indeed, most communities, suggesting that the mean intake of iodine is little more than the requirement. Under these circumstances, individuals with a greater than average requirement, e.g. rapidly growing children and young pregnant women, risk becoming deficient.

Iodine is concentrated in the thyroid gland where it is used in the synthesis of the thyroid hormones, thyroxine and triiodothyronine, and when the diet is deficient in iodine the gland enlarges to form a goitre, known also as 'Derbyshire neck' because of the prevalence of the condition in the Peak District at one time. The degree of enlargement of the thyroid depends on the extent of the deficiency and in cases of extreme deficiency the goitres are quite enormous and very disfiguring. Most 'simple' goitres (due to a primary deficiency of iodine) are not associated with any clinical symptoms but there is a serious congenital disease of children born to iodine-deficient mothers known as cretinism. In this disease there is severe mental and/or physical retardation.

The only foods that are naturally rich in iodine are 'sea foods' – fish, crustacea, shell-fish and sea weeds – and most goitrous areas are far from the sea. Drinking water makes only a small contribution to the iodine intake. Sea water itself is not rich in iodine but the plants that live in the sea have the ability to concentrate the iodine and the animals that feed upon the plants further concentrate the element. In goitrous areas, where there is a market economy, iodine deficiency may be prevented by iodizing the table salt but, where this is not feasible, injections of iodized oil have been used successfully: the beneficial results of these injections last for several years.

Zinc is another metal in which some members of particular communities are liable to become deficient. This deficiency is most prevalent in Iran and Egypt, where the staple diet of the peasant population is unleavened bread made from whole-meal wheat flour. It is often accompanied by a deficiency of iron. This diet is not particularly deficient in zinc but its high content of phytate renders the zinc and iron unavailable for absorption by forming insoluble metal phytates. Men and women suffering from a deficiency of zinc, particularly men, show retarded physical development and are known as hypogonadal dwarfs. A deficiency of zinc and of other trace elements can also occur in malabsorption syndromes and in patients maintained for long periods on intravenous nutrition. The richest dietary sources of zinc are meat, liver, egg-yolk and pulses: fruits, vegetables and 'refined' foods such as white bread, sugar, fats and oils are poor sources of the element.

A number of other minerals are essential to human health but deficiencies of elements other than those already discussed are not common and do not constitute problems of public health.

3 Problems of Over-nutrition

3.1 Obesity

Obesity is commonly held to be the most prevalent form of malnutrition in affluent societies and to constitute major medical and public health problems in these societies. This belief stemmed largely from mortality data published by life insurance companies that purported to show that over-weight people suffer an excess mortality more or less proportional to the extent to which they are over-weight. (An excess mortality of 15%, for example, means that for every 100 normal-weight people of a particular age and sex dying in any one year 115 people of the same age and sex but over-weight would die.)

There are obvious difficulties in defining what is the normal, otherwise known as 'ideal' or 'desirable' body weight and, therefore, in defining what constitutes over-weight and obesity. The best known standards for weight for height are those prepared by the Metropolitan Life Insurance Co. (U.S.A.) and these standards are for people aged 25 and over. They distinguish people of small, medium and large frame, but frame-size is not defined. Frame sizes do in fact represent the range of weights around the mean of the lower, middle and upper thirds of the insured population of the U.S.A. in their mid-twenties regardless of the fact that most normal men and women gain weight between the ages of 25 and 60. Nevertheless, it is clearly better to have a less-than-perfect standard than no standard at all and people who use this system normally use the medium frame size figures.

In recent years, more and more people working in the field of obesity have adopted another method of assessing degrees of obesity, namely, the Body Mass Index (BMI), which is calculated by dividing body weight (kg) by the square of the height (m). Thus, for example, a 1.8 m (6 ft) man weighing 75 kg (165 lb) would have a BMI of $75/(1.8)^2 = 23$. One great advantage of BMI over standard weight-for-height tables is that it enables the degree of obesity to be expressed as a single figure.

Any definition of obesity must inevitably be arbitrary and a BMI of 25 has been suggested as a guide-line value for diagnostic purposes. This value must be used sensibly and it would be foolish, for example, to say that all people with a BMI of 25.1 are obese whereas those with a BMI of 24.9 are not. However, people with a real over-weight problem have BMIs far higher than 25, e.g. 35 or 40 or greater. It has been found experimentally that almost everyone with a BMI above 25 has more than 35% fat in their bodies and that the body-fat content of nearly all people with an index below 25 is less than 35%.

The earlier data published by the insurance companies showing, for example, that men who were 10% above their ideal weight had an excess mortality of 13% have now been shown to be unreliable, mainly because the insured population providing the mortality statistics was not a true sample of the population of the country as a whole. Furthermore, where prospective policy-holders did not have a medical examination, there was no guarantee that they filled in their true body weight on the application form. Scientifically conducted prospective trials in which volunteers were studied over many years have shown that moderate degrees of over-weight unaccompanied by diabetes or hypertension (high blood pressure) are not associated with excess mortality. Serious over-weight does, however, carry with it the risk of excess mortality and since there is a tendency for obesity to increase with age and, therefore, for a mild obesity to lead on to a serious obesity, nobody who is somewhat over-weight can afford to be complacent.

Up to now, we have been equating obesity with over-weight but this is not necessarily so. The characteristic feature of obesity is the possession of excessive amounts of body fat but certain athletes, e.g. weight-lifters, are above their ideal weight for height, not because they are excessively fat but because their muscular development is abnormally great. Clearly, if one is primarily interested in body fat one should attempt to measure body fat and not body weight or body mass index. Body fat, however, is rather more difficult to measure accurately than body weight and height. The only suitable method for estimating fat on a routine basis is by measurement of skin-fold thicknesses, which measures subcutaneous fat, but which permits total body fat to be calculated. In practice, however, BMI is a perfectly acceptable index of obesity for assessing obesity in adults.

The causes of obesity   It is sometimes said that 'if you're fat you eat too much' but the nutrition scientist would want to modify this dictum by saying 'if you're fat you must, in the past, have eaten too much in relation to your energy expenditure', for it has been shown that, on average, obese people do not in fact eat more than non-obese people of the same age, sex and height.

All human beings obey the first law of thermodynamics, the law of conservation of energy, so that when the body is in energy balance the metabolisable energy (ME) derived from the food, i.e. the gross energy of the food minus the gross energy in the excreta, is equal to the energy expenditure, i.e. the energy given off from the body as heat and as the latent heat of evaporation of water. When the body is in negative energy balance, the energy expenditure is greater than the intake of ME and the extra energy is obtained by release of some of the chemical energy stored in the body as glycogen or fat. Under these conditions, there is a loss of body weight. When the energy expenditure is less than the dietary intake of ME the surplus energy is stored as fat and there is a gain in weight more or less equal to the amount of fat stored. It is this latter situation that leads to the development of obesity.

Energy expenditure is another name for heat production and the heat produced by the body and lost to the environment arises in a number of different ways, i.e. the heat of resting metabolism, the heat arising from the performance of physical work (including all muscular movement and exercise as well as 'work' in the conventional sense of the word) and the extra heat produced after eating. The technical name for the last of these components is the thermic effect of feeding, previously known as 'specific dynamic action'.

The equation for energy balance per unit of time can be expressed thus:

$ME = RM + EW + TEF + EB$ where ME = dietary intake of Metabolizable Energy; RM = Resting Metabolism; EW = Energy expended as Work; TEF = Thermic Effect of Feeding; EB = Energy Balance. When EB is positive the subject is gaining energy which, in the adult non-pregnant, non-lactating individual means gaining fat.

It is a common-place observation that some thin people eat substantially more than some overweight people of the same age, sex and height without themselves gaining weight and without engaging in any more physical exercise than their overweight counterparts. How can this paradox be explained? From the above equation it is clear that these overweight individuals must *either* have a lower RM *or* a lower TEF than the lean ones (or both). (The energy cost of a unit of work is the same in overweight as in thin people.)

Some scientists carrying out research in the field of obesity tend to stress the input side of the energy equation while others stress the output side but it is clear that both are equally important and that the only way to prevent obesity is to adjust energy intake so that it is equal to or less than the energy expenditure. There is no single cause of obesity. The simplest one, but by no means the commonest, is pure gluttony, the ingestion of amounts of food that are excessive by any standard and for these people the remedy is obvious.

Voluntary food intake is very precisely regulated in laboratory animals fed on normal diets by a number of different physiological mechanisms and whereas these mechanisms are also thought to operate in man they are all too easily over-ridden by customary eating habits and by a conscious desire to enjoy palatable foods. Laboratory rats also lose their ability to regulate their energy intake when offered particularly tasty foods instead of standard pellets. Most people are constrained to control their energy intakes far more by an awareness that their skirts or trousers are getting tight around the waist than by the operation of nervous or chemical stimuli to the appetite-controlling centres in their brain.

Let us now return to the overweight individual whose energy intake is no more and often less than normal and consider this problem in relation to RM and TEF. RM is very variable in both normal and overweight people and there is no reason to believe that the mean RM per unit of lean tissue mass differs between the two groups. However, when there is a positive energy balance over a long period, i.e. during the development of obesity, RM increases to a greater or lesser extent, and it is quite possible, therefore, that a low RM and/or one that is relatively unresponsive to a raised energy intake may contribute to obesity in individual cases. This long-term adaptation to a high energy intake is probably mediated via the thyroid gland and the sympathetic nervous system and is known as dietary induced thermogenesis (DIT).

The thermic effect of feeding has been the subject of much research in recent years and there can now be little doubt that many obese people are less able to 'burn off' excess dietary energy than normal-weight people. This effect is thought to arise partly from the increased energy expenditure resulting from the conversion of the components of the meal into body constituents and partly from the activation of specific heat-generating metabolic cycles. It is only the latter processes that appear to differ in obese and non-obese individuals.

The thermic response depends on the composition of the meal and on its size and the response reaches a plateau when large meals are taken. Whereas this plateau is reached with relatively small meals in people who do not have a weight problem and who can eat what they like without becoming fat, people with a tendency to put on weight easily respond less to small meals, although their maximum response (to large meals) is about the same as in the former group.

In summary, then, obesity arises when, over a period of time, energy intake exceeds energy expenditure, i.e. when there is a positive energy balance. The energy intake need not be high in absolute terms for this to happen but it must be high in relation to energy expenditure. A positive energy balance can thus arise because energy expenditure is below normal for any of the following reasons, alone or in combination: low RM, poor adaptation of RM to excess energy intake, low TEF and lack of exercise. Daily RM, for example, may vary by at least 4.2 MJ (1000 kcal) between two individuals of the same age, sex and body weight and the DIT resulting from a 2.1 MJ (500 kcal) meal can vary between individuals by 500 kJ (120 kcal) or more in the 4 h period after the meal; this can represent an increase over RM of up to 60%.

Obesity in infants and children   There is a widespread view that overweight infants grow into overweight children who, in turn, develop into overweight adolescents and adults, i.e. that the seeds of obesity are sown in infancy. The rationale behind this view is the belief that fat cells only develop from pre-adipocytes during infancy and that when babies are over-fed, as some artificially-fed babies tend to be, particularly if they are given solid foods at an early age, the number of fat cells in their adipose tissue increases so that their potential for storing fat and, therefore, for becoming obese, is increased. This theory has its attractions but it has now been largely discounted. Nevertheless, there can be little doubt that obesity does run in families. Epidemiological surveys have shown that there is a strong tendency for obese mothers to have overweight infants and children and that the link between obesity in fathers and children is less strong but still significant. The relative importance of 'nature' and 'nurture' in this link is not known for certain but studies with identical and non-identical twins indicates that a tendency to obesity is strongly inherited.

The food intake of infants and children varies just as much as in adults and there is little or no relationship between energy intake and obesity. Fat babies often have quite low intakes of milk and they become fat because their energy expenditure is low. Again, infants of normal weight often have prodigious appetites: presumably such infants burn off much of their dietary energy and release it as heat. In other words, RM and TEF vary in infants just as in adults.

Slimming or weight reduction   Obesity was discussed earlier in relation to the possible risk of premature death that it carries, but many people, particularly fashion-conscious women anxious to remain or become slim, regard the overweight state not as a 'health hazard' but as an unaesthetic condition that makes them unattractive to themselves and to other people. Social pressures exercised mainly by the advertising industry and by women's magazines reinforce the ideal of the slim figure that western societies hold in high esteem. The same media that exalt the slim figure tempt the appetite with multi-coloured pictures of delicious dishes, thus creating a conflict in the individual that many find hard to resolve.

The theoretical basis of weight reduction is extremely simple: it can be achieved by going into negative energy balance either by reducing energy intake or by increasing energy expenditure. The only component of energy expenditure that can readily be manipulated is the exercise component. Thus, weight reduction can be achieved either by reducing energy intake or by taking more exercise or both. This is easier said than done. There are no safe short cuts to weight reduction and any overweight persons wishing to slim and to stay slim must be prepared to work hard at it and to make permanent alterations to their dietary habits and possibly their life style. Nobody should go on a diet without familiarizing themselves with the basic principles of nutrition and without some good food tables in their hand and they should go into the enterprise with their eyes open, recognizing that it will be a long haul. It is seldom possible to reduce energy intake sufficiently solely by changing the nature of the diet and it follows, therefore, that people must eat less total food when attempting to lose weight. Eating and drinking are two of the pleasures of life and to deny oneself these pleasures requires a good deal of will-power. Furthermore, a high degree of motivation is required to put up with the pangs of hunger day after day until the body has adapted to a lower energy intake and it is not surprising that so many would-be slimmers fail to stay the course and fall by the wayside.

Requirements for protein, minerals and most vitamins are the same on a high-energy as on a reduced-energy intake. It is important, therefore, that reducing diets maintain the intake of all essential nutrients while decreasing the intake of energy. This means that the lowered energy intake should be achieved by reducing the consumption of those foods and drinks that are high in energy but low in nutrients, foods which are traditionally known as suppliers of 'empty calories'. Examples of such foods are sugar, alcoholic and soft drinks, confectionary, chocolate, ice cream, sweet biscuits, pastries and jam. It is unreasonable to make these foods completely taboo, however, as they include many that are highly palatable and the more rigid the diet the less easy it is to adhere to for long periods.

It is not wise to consume diets that are exceptionally low in energy (substantially less than the resting metabolism) for any but the shortest periods, since it is virtually impossible to obtain the minimum requirements of nutrients from such diets. Furthermore, they induce an unacceptable rate of lean tissue loss. However, very low-energy 'crash' diets probably do not harm for periods of a week or so and they enable substantial loss of weight to occur, up to 6 kg or so in a week, which may be good for the morale. However, such a rapid loss of weight is not much good for the waist-line as most of the weight loss is due to loss of water rather than fat, associated partly with a reduction in the glycogen stores and partly with a loss of soft tissue consisting largely of protein. Even quite modest reductions in energy intake will result, initially, in relatively large losses of weight, and for the same reasons.

The most commonly prescribed weight-reducing diet for an average woman is one providing 4.2 MJ (1000 kcal) and for an average man 6.3 MJ (1500 kcal). Such diets are low enough to enable most people to lose weight at a reasonable rate and high enough to supply the essential nutrients, although people with abnormally low energy expenditures may have to subsist on lower intakes than this, unless they are able to increase their expenditure by taking more exercise, e.g. by walking regularly. Again, individuals whose occupation requires them to expend large amounts of energy, may require to consume somewhat higher intakes of energy if they are to perform their work satisfactorily.

Once the glycogen reserves have been stabilized and the loss of protein halted, loss in weight on a standard reducing diet is due solely to loss in fat, which is, of course, the object of the exercise and the rate of weight loss can be calculated if the energy deficit is known. The energy content of fat-storage tissue is about 31 kJ (7.5 kcal) g^{-1} so that, for a woman with a normal energy expenditure of 8.5 MJ (2050) kcal) d^{-1}, a diet providing 4.15 MJ (1000 kcal) d^{-1} should lead theoretically to a daily weight loss of $[(8.50 - 4.15) \times 1000]/31 = 140$ g, i.e. c. 1 kg (2.25 lb) per week. This is the theoretical maximum rate of loss since the body adapts to a low energy intake by reducing RM by up to 25% and this can be the cause of much frustration in people anxious to lose weight in a hurry.

The types of food which should be avoided as far as possible by people wishing to lose weight have been mentioned above but what foods, if any, should such people be encouraged to eat? The first point that must be stressed is that there are no such foods as 'slimming' foods: it is certainly true that some foods are less energy-dense than others, i.e. they contain less energy per unit weight, but this does not help if one consumes a greater amount of the low-energy food than its normal counterpart. It is, in fact, a contradiction in terms to talk of 'slimming' foods. Incidentally, it is just as nonsensical to talk of 'fattening' foods: any food is fattening if enough is consumed.

All the foods supplying 'empty calories' are rich in either carbohydrate or fat or in both and many people anxious to reduce weight have come to regard all foods rich in fat and carbohydrate as undesirable. This is unfortunate if interpreted too literally, particularly in the case of carbohydrates, for it would mean that all starchy foods, bread, breakfast cereals, potatoes, peas and lentils, for example, would be included in the category of foods to be avoided. These foods must certainly be restricted in quantity but not banned altogether from the diet for they all contain valuable nutrients. Furthermore, a certain minimum amount of carbohydrate should be included in the diet in order to maintain normal metabolism.

Countless books and articles have been written on how to reduce weight and there are almost as many 'slimming' diets as there are authors. Their common feature, of course, is that they are all low in energy. This variety of recommended diets is all to the good, since a regimen that suits one person will not suit another. Some people find it essential for controlling their energy intake to actually weigh the major food items they consume, at least until they can judge weights accurately, and to calculate their energy intake from food tables. Others manage quite well by making a judicious selection of foods and by taking small helpings.

No attempt will be made here to present specific diet sheets but a few general suggestions – 'tips for slimmers' – may not be out of place here to summarise and augment the points made above.

1) Do not expect to lose weight at a rate greater than 0.5–1 kg (1–2 lb) week^{-1} after the initial, rapid rate of weight loss.

2) Cut down fat intake by avoiding fried foods, whole-cream cheeses, mayonnaise, fatty meat, sausage and processed meats, etc. When eating bread and cheese do without the butter.

3) If possible, give up sugar in tea and coffee and avoid sweets, chocolate, ice cream, rich desserts and other foods high in sugar such as canned fruits. (Remember that many processed foods, such as baked beans, have sugar added to them.)

4) Eat whole-meal or some other high-fibre bread rather than white bread, take one thick slice rather than several thin slices and use the minimum amount of butter or margarine. (It is foolish to replace one slice of bread by several crisp-breads, each spread with butter.)

5) Eat masses of fresh salads, fruits and vegetables in season to fill the aching void.

6) When hunger pangs become intolerable, try and assuage them with a relatively bulky food of low energy-density rather than with food of high energy density, e.g. if you are still hungry after the main course at dinner, have another helping of green vegetables rather than of potatoes: if you are hungry in between meals, eat an apple rather than a bar of chocolate or some potato crisps.

7) Remember that alcohol contains a great deal of energy.

8) Take plenty of exercise.

9) Seek support from your family and friends and possibly join a group of like-minded slimmers.

10) If you fail to lose weight at the expected rate, blame yourself rather than the first law of thermodynamics: either your energy intake is too great or your energy expenditure too little, so you must either decrease the former or increase the latter or, preferably, both at the same time.

3.2   Diseases of the cardiovascular system

There are a number of diseases of the cardiovascular system with which nutrition has been linked, namely, coronary heart disease ('heart attacks' and related conditions), hypertension (raised blood pressure) and cerebrovascular accidents ('strokes').

Coronary heart disease (CHD), otherwise known as ischaemic heart disease or, more simply, as 'heart disease', is the commonest cause of death in Britain and most other countries of the western world. This would not necessarily be a cause for concern if most of the victims were past the age of retirement but the most worrying aspect of the problem is that the disease afflicts many men in their prime of life and in Britain more and more men in the 30–55 age group are dying of CHD. There is no single cause of CHD and many factors play a part in its development. Among the most important of these so-called 'risk factors' are smoking, hypertension, elevated levels of plasma lipids and diabetes. Stress, lack of exercise and serious obesity are also accepted as risk factors and there can be little doubt that there is a genetic component to the disease. Up until the age of about 50, the great majority of the victims of CHD are men but from this age onwards an increasing number of women die of the disease. It is considered, therefore, that reproductive steroids influence the development of CHD, although their precise role is not clear. The simplest explanation is either that androgens are atherogenic and/or thrombogenic or that oestrogens exert a protective action, but the situation is almost certainly more complicated than this.

CHD expresses itself in a number of different ways (i) *Angina pectoris*: this is typified by serious chest pains brought on by exercise or by emotional stress. In this condition, the coronary arteries are unable to supply sufficient oxygen to the heart muscle to enable it to perform the extra work required of it. (ii) *Myocardial infarction*: this is the condition that results from a heart attack. The blood supply to part of the heart muscle is interrupted by a blockage in a branch of a coronary artery and the affected muscle tissue becomes ischaemic (starved of blood) and dies. The severity of a myocardial infarction depends on the area of heart muscle affected; it may or may not be fatal. (iii) *Sudden death*: this may occur as a result of myocardial infarction or of a cardiac arrest due to ventricular fibrillation caused by a disruption of the normal pathways of electrical conduction of the heart.

All of these conditions have a common origin, namely, the arterial disease known as atherosclerosis. In this disease there is a narrowing of the arteries brought about by a thickening of the arterial wall by a proliferation of smooth muscle-like cells and by an accumulation of fatty material. Atherosclerosis alone will not induce a heart attack but it may give rise to angina. For a heart attack to occur the restricted lumen of one of the branches of a coronary artery must be occluded by a thrombus, a mass of clotted blood that forms over an ulcerated atherosclerotic lesion affecting the wall of the artery. There are, thus, two major components of CHD, atherosclerosis and thrombosis, and both are influenced by diet.

The early development of atherosclerosis is associated with damage to the endothelial lining of arteries and one way in which the initial injury to the arterial wall may be induced is by thrombus formation. Thrombosis may thus have a role in both the initial and the final stages of CHD.

Atherosclerosis   The major link between nutrition and atherosclerosis is one involving the plasma concentration of low-density lipoproteins (LDL), the major cholesterol-carrying fraction of the blood lipids, which is readily influenced by diet. Epidemiological studies have shown that there is a close relationship between the mean concentration of LDL cholesterol in a population and the incidence of CHD. Since, the high-density lipoproteins (HDL) of the plasma appear to exert a protective action against CHD, the ratios of total cholesterol or LDL cholesterol to HDL cholesterol are better indices of the likely incidence of CHD in a population than the concentration of LDL cholesterol. Raised levels of plasma triglycerides also constitute a risk factor for CHD.

The theory relating diet to CHD that has received the greatest attention is the 'saturated fat' theory, but before discussing this theory brief consideration must be given to the different types of fats present in the diet. Saturated fats are fats that are rich in saturated fatty acids and they are solid at room temperatures.

Typical examples are the milk and depot fats of ruminant animals and coconut oil. In terms of actual foods, those high in saturated fats include butter, hard margarine and shortenings, suet and foods prepared from these fats, e.g. pastry and ice cream: full cream cheeses, beef and lamb are other sources.

All unsaturated fatty acids and lipids containing large amounts of these acids are liquid at room temperature. The commonest monounsaturated acid is oleic acid, which is widely distributed in fats and oils and which is particularly abundant in olive oil. There are two main families of polyunsaturated fatty acids, the, so-called, n–3 and n–6 series, and these acids include the essential fatty acids which cannot be synthesised in the body and which must therefore be supplied in the diet. The n–3 series are particularly abundant in fish oils and they are present in small concentrations in many other foods. (Linseed oil contains large amounts of one particular acid of this series, α-linolenic acid, but this oil is not normally consumed by man.) The most abundant fatty acid of the n–6 series present in dietary fats is linoleic acid: most cooking and salad oils, e.g. corn, soya, sunflower and groundnut oils, (but not olive oil) are particularly rich in this acid and so are many soft margarines.

The 'saturated fat' theory relates diet to CHD, according to which a high intake of saturated fat constitutes an important risk factor for CHD. Some of the main arguments commonly brought forward in support of this theory are as follows:

1) Epidemiological studies have shown that there are close links between (a) the mean plasma concentration of total cholesterol (a rough index of LDL cholesterol), (b) the intake of saturated fat and (c) the incidence of CHD in a population.

2) In experimental animals, plasma cholesterol levels and the degree of atherosclerosis are increased by diets rich in saturated fat and these effects are reduced when the saturated fat (S) is replaced by polyunsaturated fat (P).

3) In man, too, levels of plasma cholesterol can be reduced by increasing the P:S ratio of the dietary fat and in a number of primary prevention trials in which the diet was altered in this way the incidence of CHD was reduced.

4) In men, forty years of age, mortality from CHD is almost three times as great in Edinburgh as in Stockholm and the fatty acids of the adipose tissue, which reflect the long-term composition of the diet, have a significantly higher P:S ratio in the Swedish men that in the Scots.

5) In Belgium, the incidence of CHD is higher in the south than in the north of the country, associated with a mean dietary P:S ratio of 0.19 in the butter-eating south and a ratio of 0.42 in the margarine-eating north.

These pieces of evidence are highly selective and they relate primarily to the atherosclerosis component of CHD. This is the main weakness of the 'saturated fat' theory; it ignores the involvement of thrombosis and of heart muscle function in the manifestation of the disease. Within any high-risk population there is no correlation between dietary intakes of saturated fatty acids and plasma cholesterol in individuals. Furthermore, when different high-risk populations are compared, there are no significant differences between the severity and extent of atherosclerosis in moderately high- and very high-risk communities. Whereas the main difference between populations with high and low incidences of CHD is almost certainly in the extent of atherosclerosis, it may well be that the difference in mortality from CHD between different high-risk populations is related more to variations in the clotting properties of the blood and to the reaction of the myocardium to abnormal stimuli than to variations in the extent of arterial disease.

Diets high in saturated fatty acids are, almost inevitably, low in poly-unsaturated fatty acids and it has been suggested that it is a *deficiency* of polyunsaturated, rather than an *excess* of saturated, fatty acids that constitutes a serious risk factor for CHD. However, a more balanced view is that both factors are important.

Thrombosis Polyunsaturated fatty acids (PUFA) are present in large amounts in cholesterol esters and in phospholipids, which means that they have an important role in lipid transport and in membrane function. They also affect the clotting properties of the blood. The most striking evidence for this involvement in blood clotting comes from a study of Greenland Eskimos. The incidence of CHD is very low in these people and their blood shows an exceptionally low clotting ability, so much so that they experience frequent nose-bleeds. This low tendency of the blood to clot is associated with abnormal platelet function: aggregation of the blood platelets is an important step in thrombus formation and the platelets of Eskimos aggregate poorly. Experiments with human volunteers have shown that platelet aggregation can be reduced to the low level observed in Eskimos within a week or so by the consumption of large amounts of oily fish. A specific PUFA of the n–3 series, eicosapentaenoic acid (EPA), is responsible for this alteration in platelet activity and all oily fish and oils such as cod-liver oil are rich sources of EPA. The extent to which other dietary PUFA of the n–3 series, such as α-linolenic acid, might be able to fulfil the role of EPA itself, either by conversion to this acid or by some other mechanism, is not clear but it is a reasonable possibility. However, the 'classical' essential fatty acids of the n–6 series, linoleic and arachidonic, certainly cannot be converted to EPA.

The role of PUFA in platelet aggregation is exceedingly complex. Furthermore, it is a field in which knowledge is advancing very rapidly, so that any detailed scheme that might be formulated today would be likely to be out of date in a few months time. Suffice it to say that PUFA of the n–3 and n–6 series containing twenty carbon atoms give rise to prostaglandin-like substances some of which are pro- and some anti- aggregatory and that an important factor in determining the tendency to thrombus formation is the balance between the n–3, n–6 series of PUFA.

The exaggerated reduction in platelet aggregation observed in Eskimos carries with it an increased risk of a serious haemorrhage, e.g. in child-birth, but a modest reduction in platelet aggregability in populations with a high risk of CHD would seem to be wholly desirable.

Dietary PUFA also influence plasma lipid concentrations, as noted earlier, but most of the research that was carried out on this aspect of nutrition took place before the full significance of the different metabolic roles of the n–3 and n–6 PUFA was realised. Consequently, all the different PUFA were added together in calculating P:S ratios. However, it should be noted that acids of the n–6 series always predominate in western diets and that the n–6 : n–3 ratio for most European diets ranges between 5 and 10.

Myocardial arrhythmias   The possible role of fatty acids in the ventricular fibrillation that sometimes develops during the acute ischaemic phase of a heart attack is still a matter of uncertainty but it is possible that certain mixtures of fatty acids liberated from triglycerides as a result of catecholamine release may interfere with the normal propagation of the nerve impulses that control the contraction of the heart muscle. Nervous conduction depends on the movement of cations across membranes which in turns depends on the maintenance of normal ion gradients on either side of the membranes, so that any disturbance in these gradients may cause arrhythmias in the heart. Sodium, potassium, calcium and magnesium ions all play essential roles in normal neuro-muscular function, and in this connection, interest has focussed more on the last two of these ions, both of which combine with free fatty acids.

Other dietary risk factors for CHD   Epidemiological studies have indicated that vegetarian diets and ones high in dietary fibre may exert some protective action against CHD and, conversely, that diets rich in animal products (meat, butter, cheese, in particular) and low in fibre constitute risk factors for CHD. The results of other studies have shown that moderate intakes of alcohol increase high density lipoprotein levels in the blood, thereby reducing the risk of CHD. Heavy drinkers, however, run an *increased* risk of CHD. A number of investigations have shown that high intakes of sucrose are associated with high rates of CHD but this may be because there is a strong correlation between the intake of saturated fat and the intake of sucrose in many western societies. However, when the effects of other dietary variables are eliminated by suitable statistical techniques, the residual association between sucrose intake and CHD is weak.

The mechanisms by which diets high in fibre and in plant proteins influence the risk of CHD is not entirely clear but there is experimental evidence that plant proteins and some types of dietary fibre have a hypocholesterolaemic action.

In Britain, the incidence of CHD is higher in areas where the drinking water is soft than in hard-water areas. A number of suggestions have been made to explain the role of soft water in increasing the risk of CHD, e.g. excess of toxic elements, deficiency of magnesium and other essential minerals, but there is no good experimental evidence to support these ideas. It seems probable that hardness of water relates more to myocardial function than to atherosclerosis or thrombosis.

Dietary cholesterol has been considered as a risk factor for CHD, partly from epidemiological studies and partly from experiments in which experimental animals have been fed on diets high in cholesterol. Such diets certainly cause a type of atherosclerosis in some species but it presents a different histological picture from the one observed in natural atherosclerosis in man. Human diets rich in cholesterol are normally rich in saturated fatty acids as well and it now appears unlikely that dietary cholesterol is an independent risk factor for CHD.

Coronary prevention   Any realistic policy for reducing the incidence of CHD in a population or for reducing the risk of CHD in a particular individual must recognize the multi-factorial nature of the disease and should tackle all the risk factors that can readily be modified. Risk factors are additive and they may interact with and amplify one another, so that attempts to reduce any risk factors are worth while. It is by no means certain that nutrition is the most important risk factor: smoking and hypertension, for example, appear to be more important than diet in increasing the risk of a heart attack in western societies and although the evidence is not particularly strong, it seems probable that lack of exercise may also be a significant risk factor.

This having been said, however, and since this is a book on nutrition, the possibility of reducing the risk of CHD by dietary means must be considered seriously. It is highly probable that the incidence of CHD in the affluent industrial societies of the west would decrease markedly if we adopted the diets consumed by the rural populations of, say, India or Africa, which consist largely of cereals and pulses with only small amounts of animal products and sugar. However, it would be completely unrealistic to suppose that a drastic change of this nature could be brought about in entire populations although it would not be difficult for individuals to alter their diet in this way if they are sufficiently motivated. (It is perhaps worth mentioning here that, except where religious prohibitions apply, people everywhere in poor countries aspire to the western type of diet rich in animal products, and adopt such a diet whenever economic circumstances permit. CHD is, indeed, a disease of affluence.)

The aim, therefore, should be to modify the diet rather than to revolutionize it and for normal healthy individuals and populations the best recommendation is that they should simply 'follow the principles of good nutrition'. The most important of these principles is that the diet should be as varied as possible, i.e. should comprise a wide range of different foods. This minimizes the risk of any one nutrient being in excess or in deficit. The cumulative evidence that an excessive intake of fat, particularly saturated fat, is undesirable is too great for it to be ignored and any prudent diet should recognize this fact. There is now a large degree of consensus among nutritionists that fat should not provide more than about 35% of the total energy intake. By simply reducing the intake of total fat the P:S ratio of the diet will almost inevitably increase but this ratio can be increased further in quite a simple manner by substituting oils such as corn or soyabean oil for lard and other solid fats in frying and by partially replacing butter by a polyunsaturated margarine. The outcome of obtaining fat from a wide variety of sources – oil seeds, cereals, fish, butter, eggs, margarine and meat – and of consuming these fats, together with a good mixture of other foods – cereals, pulses, fruits, vegetables and poultry meat – is 'a good mixed diet'. Finally, the reader might like to refer back to the list of recommendations given for those wishing to lose weight (pp. 30–31), many of which are relevant in the present context.

Hypertension   In affluent societies the blood pressure of most individuals rises progressively with age but in many undeveloped countries this rise does not occur. Thus, hypertension would appear to be related in some way to life-style: there is also a strong genetic component.

A high intake of sodium relative to potassium has long been considered to be the major dietary factor contributing to hypertension and the epidemiological evidence linking salt intake with hypertension is very strong. However, recent research has shown that individuals vary widely in their susceptibility to salt-induced hypertension: whereas some are quite sensitive to a continuous high intake of salt others are relatively insensitive. Nevertheless, a high-salt diet is of no positive benefit to anyone, except perhaps in tropical countries where substantial losses of salt occur in the sweat and it is common sense to restrict one's salt intake. A taste for salt is as easy to lose as to acquire.

In western countries, the mean blood pressure of vegetarians is less than that of non-vegetarians. There is experimental evidence that high-fat diets increase blood pressure and that diets high in fibre reduce it and since vegetarians' diets tend to be low in fat and salt and high in fibre, all of these dietary factors may contribute to the overall result.

Obesity and hypertension frequently go together and blood pressure often falls when a weight-reducing regimen is followed. Mild hypertension need not be a cause for concern but serious hypertension is an important risk-factor for CHD and for cerebrovascular accidents and people who do not respond to diet require to be treated with hypotensive drugs.

Cerebrovascular accidents (strokes)   The role of diet in the aetiology of cerebrovascular disease is not at all clear. Both CHD and cerebrovascular disease develop against a background of arterial disease and both are exacerbated by hypertension but here the parallel ends. The death rate from strokes has not increased significantly during the last fifty years, in contrast to the astronomical increase in deaths from CHD over this period. Furthermore, men and women are equally affected. Cerebrovascular disease is not particularly common until the age of about 65: after this age, it is one of the commonest causes of death. Strokes are caused by an interruption of the blood supply to the brain brought about either by haemorrhage of a diseased artery or by occlusion of an artery by a clot of blood developing *in situ* or transported to the brain from elsewhere in the body. The severity of a stroke depends on the area of the brain affected and on the length of time that elapses before a collateral circulation is established. Ischaemia can also occur without the occlusion of an artery, solely because of the temporary inability of the diseased arteries to carry sufficient blood to the brain.

It is generally agreed that hypertension is the major factor that predisposes to cerebrovascular accidents and any link that may exist between nutrition and cerebrovascular disease is probably mediated by way of the effect of nutrition on blood pressure. However, the link between nutrition and hypertension and cere-brovascular disease is much less strong than that between nutrition and CHD.

3.3   Diabetes mellitus

Is a disease of metabolism brought about either by a failure of the body to produce sufficient insulin or of the tissues to respond normally to the hormone. Metabolism of carbohydrate, protein and fat are all impaired. Two major types of diabetes are recognized, juvenile-onset and maturity-onset: the former type normally develops by the age of 10 or 12 but its appearance is occasionally delayed until the thirties; the latter type develops in middle age after the age of forty. Both types have a strong hereditary element but environmental factors determine whether or not genetically predisposed individuals actually develop the disease. Nutrition is a major environmental factor in the development of maturity-onset diabetes and it plays a vital role in the management of the disease. Most maturity-onset diabetics are obese. At one time it was thought that diabetes was induced by excessive consumption of carbohydrates, particularly of sugar, but it is now recognized that the true predisposing factor is an excessive intake of energy in whatever form it is ingested.

Management of all cases of juvenile-onset diabetes requires some form of insulin to be administered regularly but the disease can be controlled in most maturity-onset diabetics either by diet alone or by a combination of diet and oral hypoglycaemic drugs. The treatment of diabetes by dietary means is a vast subject best dealt with in books devoted to clinical nutrition or dietetics but some of the general principles can appropriately be considered here.

For obese diabetics a major requirement is to prescribe a weight-reducing diet following the principles noted earlier (pp. 30–31). Once a normal weight has been achieved, the main aim must be to control the level of blood sugar, since most of the secondary complications of diabetes are the result of hyperglycaemia (an elevated concentration of glucose in the blood), and, indeed, this aim must also be borne in mind during the weight-reducing phase of diabetic control, for it is of paramount importance. In western societies, the traditional way in which people have sought to control the blood sugar of diabetics by diet has been by restricting the intake of carbohydrate and by ensuring that food is consumed in regular amounts and at regular intervals throughout the day to minimize the fluctuations in blood sugar. The classical 'diabetic' diet is thus low in carbohydrate and, inevitably, high in fat: in other words, it is what is now commonly regarded as an atherogenic diet. It is well known that the death rate from CHD is very high among diabetics in western communities and it is not sensible, therefore, needlessly to increase the risk of CHD inherent in the diabetic state.

Diabetics in countries of the Far East, such as India and Japan, have long been successfully managed by diets high in carbohydrates and the traditional western diabetic diet is being increasingly questioned. It is accepted that soluble sugars should be restricted because of the rapidity with which the products of their digestion are absorbed into the blood but foods rich in complex carbohydrates, including starch, are now looked upon more favourably, although the requirement for meals to be regular remains in the prescription.

Dietary fibre is very useful in the management of diabetes; it slows down the rate of digestion and absorption of carbohydrates thereby lowering the post-prandial peak in the concentration of blood sugar. Certain gums, e.g. guar gum, are particularly effective in exerting this action and they have been used therapeutically in the dietary control of diabetes. Guar gum comes from the seed of a leguminous plant and legumes such as lentils, soyabeans and chick peas are excellent foods for diabetics because their carbohydrates are digested and absorbed much slower than the carbohydrates of cereals.

4 Other Disorders with a Nutritional Component

4.1 Food allergies and intolerances

Some people experience unpleasant symptoms of varying intensity when they eat particular foods and when these symptoms have an immunological origin the reactions are known as allergies. When the mechanism is non-immunological the diseases are referred to as food intolerances and they are mainly caused by hereditary deficiencies in specific enzymes. One of the commonest examples is lactose intolerance.

Food allergies show themselves in various ways: physical reactions include asthma, skin rash, eczema, headache, migraine, abdominal pain, vomiting and diarrhoea but mental symptoms such as depression and schizophrenia have also been reported. There is evidence, too, that some behavioural problems in children, characterized by hyper-activity, may also be caused by food allergies. Some foods are more likely to induce allergies than others: wheat, eggs and milk provoke allergies more frequently than any other foods but almost any food is capable of causing an adverse reaction in particular individuals. Proteins are most frequently responsible but artificial colours, flavouring agents and preservatives are also potentially allergenic.

For a foreign substance to provoke an immune reaction it must gain entrance to the body via one of the mucosal surfaces, usually the gut or the lungs. It used to be thought that dietary proteins are completely broken down to amino acids in the digestive tract but it is now recognized that small amounts of undegraded and partially degraded proteins are absorbed across the gut as a normal feature of the digestive process. Any such foreign molecules (known as antigens) may provoke an immune response, i.e. induce the formation of antibodies: this is part of the normal mechanism by which the body protects itself against toxins and other potentially harmful substances. Allergies arise when this response, normally beneficial, expresses itself in an abnormal manner.

One of the ways in which animals protect themselves from the harmful immunological effects of dietary proteins is by secreting antibodies to these proteins in the intestinal mucous. The resulting antigen-antibody complex is then digested by proteolytic enzymes. If the amount of antigen, i.e. the dietary protein, is greatly in excess of the antibody secreted by the intestinal mucosa, some of the protein may become attached to antibodies located on the surface of mast cells present in the mucosal layer and stimulate them to secrete pharmacologically active substances which cause inflammation and tissue damage. In the gut release of these substances produces symptoms such as abdominal pain, vomiting or diarrhoea.

Most normal people have antibodies to a whole variety of common foods circulating in their blood plasma and these circulating antibodies protect the body by combining with their particular antigens to give a complex which is normally removed from the circulation by phagocytes. If, however, the circulating antibodies are overwhelmed by the quantity of antigen absorbed, molecules of the latter may attach themselves to antibodies located in the tissues and trigger off the release of vaso-active amines. If the tissue involved is the lung, the allergy expresses itself in the form of breathlessness or even asthma; if the antibodies are present in the skin, a nettle rash or eczema develops. When migraine is brought on by the consumption of particular foods or drinks, it may be due to the presence of a pharmacologically-active agent in the food altering the blood flow in the brain: on the other hand, the migraine may be a true allergy in which the active substances responsible are produced in the brain itself as a result of an immune reaction.

Food allergies are more common in infants and young children than in older children and adults, possibly due to immaturity of the digestive or immune systems. Cows' milk allergy is the commonest type and considering the huge antigenic load to which artificially-fed infants are subjected this is not, perhaps, surprising. Eczema and/or gastro-intestinal pains are the usual symptoms. Risk of this disorder is minimized by exclusive breast feeding for as long as possible but occasionally the antigen is transmitted in breast milk from the diet of the mother. In serious cases of this allergy, milk-substitutes based on soya bean proteins must be given instead of cows' milk and some infants then become hypersensitive to soya protein. Indeed, it is a general observation that most individuals, both young and adult, that suffer from food allergy are sensitive to a number of different foods and many of these individuals are also susceptible to other types of allergy, e.g. to pollen, house dust and animals. A generalized hypersensitivity to foreign substances in the environment is known as atopy and it is a familial disorder, i.e. it is genetic in origin.

It is usually possible to identify the offending food when the adverse effects occur immediately after it is consumed but when the effects are delayed, as is so often the case, it is very difficult to pin-point the food or foods responsible. Blood and skin tests are not satisfactory for diagnosing food allergies, and the only reliable way of diagnosing a particular condition as a case of genuine food allergy is by demonstrating unequivocally that the symptoms disappear when particular items of food are removed from the diet and re-appear when these items are once more consumed. This is not always easy to arrange in practice, especially when a large number of different foods appears to be involved. The basic idea, however, is simple: the individual is placed on a simple 'exclusion' diet free of all the common foods known to cause allergy and based on, for example, rice, sago and fresh fruits and vegetables, until the symptoms disappear. Other foods such as bread, meat, fish, eggs, milk, cheese, etc. are then added singly and sufficient time is allowed after each addition for symptoms to re-appear. These tests should be carried out under expert supervision to make sure that the subject does not develop malnutrition by remaining too long on exclusion diets which, by their very nature, are nutritionally incomplete. Particular care should be taken not to experiment in this way with the diet of infants and young children except under medical supervision.

Steatorrhoea   There are a number of diseases of the digestive tract typified by a failure to digest the food and/or to absorb the products of digestion and some of the most important of these disease conditions are considered in this section. Perhaps the commonest way in which these diseases express themselves is by the presence of excess fat in the faeces, a condition known as steatorrhoea. This may be due to a failure of pancreatic secretion, which occurs when the pancreas is diseased, or to a deficiency of biliary secretion, as in obstructive jaundice, since both pancreative lipase and bile salts are required for the normal digestion and absorption of fats. Steatorrhoea may also occur after gastro-intestinal surgery. When there is a failure of fat absorption the fat-soluble vitamins are poorly absorbed also and deficiencies of these vitamins are liable to occur when the steatorrhoea is of long standing. When the specific cause of the fat malabsorption is not amenable to treatment, a low-fat diet must be given. Short and medium chain triglycerides containing fatty acids with between 4 and 10 carbon atoms are digested and absorbed more readily than long chain triglycerides in conditions of pancreatic insufficiency. Milk fat is the richest source of short-chain fatty acids and the fats that make it up are, therefore, the ones most suitable for inclusion in the diet of people who have difficulty in absorbing fats. Medium chain triglycerides obtained from coconut oil are available for special diets.

Steatorrhoea also occurs in coeliac disease due to a failure, not to digest but to absorb fat. Indeed, there is a failure of absorption of most nutrients in this disease which is characterized by atrophy of the villi of the small intestines. This atrophy is induced by a particular protein, gliadin, soluble in 70% alcohol and found in the gluten fraction of most cereals, including wheat, rye, oats and barley and the disease is sometimes described as one of gluten intolerance. The mechanism of this sensitivity to gluten is not fully understood but it is probably of immunological origin.

Before 1950, when the cause of coeliac disease was identified, children suffering from the disease frequently died of what amounted to starvation. It is now treated by a gluten-free diet, which has to be adhered to for life. Rice and maize (corn) are the only cereals that can be tolerated, although gluten-free flour is available at a price. Great care must be taken in avoiding processed foods which contain wheat products particularly as many factory-made soups, sausages and other meat products, hamburgers, spreads, salad dressings, pudding mixes, baked beans and milk beverages contain wheat flour. Untreated coeliacs often suffer from anaemia due to defective absorption of iron, folic acid or both.

Lactose intolerance   Many people in the world, both adults and children, develop intestinal pains and diarrhoea when they drink a large glass of milk. These intestinal disturbances result from a failure to digest the lactose in the milk and the condition is known as lactose intolerance. Lactose is a disaccharide and it cannot be absorbed until it has been hydrolysed by a specific lactose-splitting enzyme located in the brush border of the cells of the small intestine. In lactose intolerance, this enzyme is permanently lost a variable time after weaning, certainly by the age of ten or twelve. When the lactose enters the large intestine it increases the osmotic pressure exerted by the intestinal contents and draws water from the blood: the lactose is fermented by lactic bacteria to give faeces of high acidity.

Lactose intolerance is much more common in some ethnic groups than in others: most peoples of African and Asian origin show a very high incidence but the members of some pastoral tribes in Africa, for whom milk forms a regular part of their diet, retain the ability to digest lactose right throughout life. Taking the human population of the world as a whole, it would appear that lactose-intolerance is more normal that lactose-tolerance. Thus, the British are abnormal in that over 90% of them retain the ability to digest large amounts of lactose.

Lactose-intolerant individuals can digest moderate amounts of lactose by virtue of intracellular lactases present within the intestinal mucosa and the prevalence of this condition in developing countries should not be allowed to restrict the use of dried milk in food-aid programmes for malnourished children.

Congenital deficiencies of lactose and of other brush-border disaccharidases occur rarely in infants from birth.

4.2 Dental caries (dental decay)

This is one of the commonest infectious diseases of man. It is more prevalent in industrial than in peasant societies and when people in developing countries acquire the dietary habits of western nations their dental health declines rapidly. Dental decay is brought about by the activity of specific bacteria that inhabit the mouth. These bacteria attach themselves to the surfaces of the teeth in association with an insoluble bacterial polysaccharide composed mainly of dextran. The complex of bacteria and polysaccharide is known as dental plaque. The bacteria produce organic acids from the fermentable carbohydrates of the food and these acids attack the teeth producing the cavities we all dread. There is an abundance of evidence that sucrose (produced from both sugar cane and sugar beet) is the most cariogenic of all carbohydrates, although other sugars and even cooked starch, have been shown to encourage tooth decay in experimental animals and they may also do so in man. Not only is sucrose more cariogenic, weight for weight, than other sugars but it is the sugar that is present in the greatest abundance in western diets. It appears to act both by stimulating plaque-forming bacteria and by providing a good substrate for the production of organic acids. From the point of view of tooth decay, sugar taken in solution, e.g. in tea and coffee, and with meals, e.g. in cakes and ice-cream, seems to be somewhat less of a risk than sugar eaten between meals in the form of snacks such as chocolate biscuits and confectionary. The major factor seems to be the length of time that the teeth are exposed to sugar, although the nature of the food is also important. Sticky foods such as chocolates and toffees are retained between the teeth and allow more time for acid-producing bacteria to work than when the sugar is in a soluble or non-sticky form.

The most important steps that the individual can take to limit dental decay are to brush the teeth regularly to remove plaque, to restrict the intake of foods rich in sugar, particularly between meals, and to avoid sticky confections as a regular part of the diet. Thus, the prescription for dental health coincides with that for good nutrition, namely, the limitation of 'empty calories' in the form of sucrose.

The teeth of some individuals are more susceptible to decay than those of others and part of this susceptibility is genetic in origin. The nutritional status of the body during tooth formation is also important. Calcium, phosphorus and vitamin D are essential for the calcification of teeth just as they are for the calcification of bones and of these nutrients vitamin D is the only one which is likely to be deficient. There is a danger, therefore, that teeth developing during a period when a child is suffering from rickets will be more susceptible to decay than normal.

Teeth that are exposed to small amounts of fluoride during development acquire some measure of resistance to caries. The nature of this resistance is not fully understood but the bacteriostatic action of the fluoride may play a part. Another factor that is probably involved is the lattice structure of the enamel crystals. These are made of the mineral apatite: fluoro-apatite crystals have a more perfect lattice structure than hydroxyapatite, the normal tooth mineral, and they fit together very precisely to give a structure more resistant to attack by acid.

Most of the fluoride in the diet is obtained from drinking water, although tea is also a good source. Among foods, sea-foods are the only ones that provide significant amounts of fluoride. Exhaustive studies have established beyond doubt that the incidence of dental caries is substantially less in areas where the drinking water contains $0.5-1$ mg l^{-1} (parts per million) fluoride than in areas, otherwise similar, where only traces of fluoride are present in the water. The protection against dental decay is observed primarily in children whose teeth have calcified under the influence of fluoride but the protective influence persists throughout life. The benefits of fluoride on teeth that have already erupted are somewhat doubtful but application of a solution of a soluble fluoride to individual teeth can reduce their susceptibility to tooth decay. There is some evidence that moderate intakes of fluoride confer to the skeleton some resistance against osteoporosis.

Some natural water supplies contain protective concentrations of fluoride and in many communities throughout the world in which the natural fluoride content is very low fluoride is added by the water authority to bring the level up to 1 mg l^{-1}. Some people object to the fluoridation of public water supplies either in the belief that fluoride constitutes a health hazard or on the ground that fluoridation of public water supplies constitutes a fundamental infringement of the basic rights of the individual. Fluoride is certainly toxic when taken in excess but millions of people throughout the world have for many years been drinking water to which fluoride has been added at a level of 1 mg l^{-1} without any untoward effects but with significant benefit to their dental health. On average, fluoridation reduces the rate of tooth decay in children by about 50%, with a range varying between 40 and 70% in different communities.

In some parts of the world, e.g. in the Arabian Gulf and in parts of India and China, very high concentrations of fluoride occur in the natural waters. The permanent teeth, particularly the upper incisors, of people who drink water containing $3-5$ mg fluoride l^{-1} during the period of tooth development become pitted and mottled with a brown pigment. Their general health is not affected in any way. (However, after prolonged exposure to drinking water containing more than 10 mg fluoride l^{-1} the skeleton may be seriously affected.)

4.3   Cancer

The different types of cancer show great variations in their incidence from country to country, which suggests that environmental factors play a major role in their development and it has been estimated that these factors are probably responsible for $c.$ 90% of human cancers. Since man has ways and means of altering the environment, if he chooses so to do, it follows that he should be able to reduce the incidence of cancer, once the environmental risk factors have been identified. Contrary to popular opinion, when deaths from lung cancer, which is primarily due to cigarette smoking, are excluded, mortality resulting from malignant diseases in the United Kingdom and in the U.S.A. is slightly less today than at the beginning of the century. It is known that many chemicals are capable of inducing cancer when applied to the skin, breathed in through the lungs or taken into the digestive tract and these substances are known as carcinogens. The great variations from country to country in the incidence of tumours of the digestive tract strongly suggest that the diet is involved. This does not necessarily mean that dietary carcinogens are the cause of these tumours: for example, intestinal bacteria may produce carcinogens from components either of the diet or of the bile. Evidence of a link between diet and the different types of cancer is largely based on epidemiological studies, i.e. on correlations between the incidence of particular cancers and specific dietary components in different populations, and such studies can never prove causal relationships. They can, however, point the way towards more direct investigations that might prove fruitful and in a few cases the epidemological evidence has been supported by clinical studies and is sufficiently strong to make a causal relationship seem likely. In most cases, however, the evidence is circumstantial and often conflicting and quite insufficient to make it possible or desirable to recommend dietary changes at the present time. This having been said, research on possible links between diet and malignant disease must be continued and extended.

The particular cancers that have been most convincingly linked with diet are cancers of the oesophagus and stomach. Epidemiological evidence strengthened by case-control studies have shown that in some populations excess consumption of alcohol is associated with an increased risk of oesophageal cancer and that this risk is greater in smokers than in non-smokers. (In case-control studies dietary intake data for patients and appropriate control subjects are compared.) In other populations alcohol is certainly not the cause of this cancer: in some parts of Iran, where the incidence of oesophageal cancer is extremely high, the people are Muslims and neither drink nor smoke. The environmental factor that determines the development of this cancer in Iran is unknown.

In the period between 1955 and 1972 there was a strong positive correlation between mortality from stomach cancer and from cerebrovascular accidents in many different countries. This correlation has been less good since 1972, probably because the improved drug treatments for hypertension introduced about this time were effective in reducing strokes but had no influence on gastric cancer. The common factor linking cerebrovascular accidents and gastric cancer is probably salt, which increases blood pressure in susceptible individuals (pp. 36–7), the mechanisms by which a high intake of salt induces cancer of the stomach is not known with any certainty but a number of different mechanisms have been proposed, e.g. by an osmotic effect causing irritation of the gastric mucosa or by delaying stomach emptying thereby prolonging contact between the mucosa and carcinogens, such as nitroso-amines, in the food. The salt hypothesis was tested in a nation-wide trial in Belgium between 1966 and 1979 in which people were encouraged by a huge publicity campaign to decrease their dietary intake of salt. This campaign was successful in reducing the mean salt intake by about 40% and a marked decrease in both strokes and gastric cancer was observed during this period.

Other associations between diet and cancer that have been suggested are ones between a low fibre intake and cancer of the large bowel and a high fat intake and cancer of the colon, breast, ovary and endometrium of the uterus. Recent evidence suggests that the severe constipation frequently experienced by people consuming a low fibre diet may provide a clue to these associations. It is known that the bacterial flora of the large intestine can transform sterols and fatty acids into a variety of carcinogens and mutagens which can be absorbed into the blood and taken up by the tissues and the longer the food residues remain in the large intestine the greater are the amounts of toxic substances that are likely to be produced.

There is evidence from an epidemiological study that the intake of β-carotene is inversely related to the incidence of lung cancer in middle-aged men, i.e. that a high intake of carotene protects against this type of cancer (but not against other cancers). It has also been suggested that increased intakes of vitamin C exert a measure of protection against some malignant diseases but at the present time the evidence is not sufficiently convincing for it to be generally accepted.

There are misgivings in the public mind that some food additives may be carcinogenic but the safeguards and testing procedures that have been established to prevent harmful substances from being added to foods are extremely stringent and public fears are quite unjustified. Naturally-occurring toxic substances are much more hazardous to health, not perhaps in affluent societies but certainly in underdeveloped populations. The best known natural carcinogen is aflatoxin, a toxin produced by certain strains of the mould *Aspergillus flavus* which may attack groundnuts (peanuts) and occasionally other foods stored in damp conditions after harvesting. This toxin was discovered following the outbreak of a new and serious disease of young turkeys and ducklings in England in 1960, during which *c.* 100 000 turkey poults died. Aflatoxin is one of the most toxic substances known to man and it may well be responsible for the high incidence of liver cancer in Thailand and in parts of Africa.

Cancer relates to nutrition in other ways: many patients suffering from malignant diseases lose weight and become severely malnourished, particularly when the digestive tract is involved.

5 Nutrition of Vulnerable Groups

In this context the term 'vulnerable' is used to describe those groups that are at particular risk of malnutrition primarily because they have a high requirement for nutrients and because their potential problems can be avoided by good nutrition. Groups that are vulnerable to malnutrition for other reasons, e.g. alcoholics and sufferers from coeliac disease, are not included.

5.1 Pregnant and nursing women

Pregnancy is a natural physiological state and during the course of evolution adaptive mechanisms have developed to protect the foetus from the harmful effects of adverse environmental factors, including the erratic supply of food. Protection against malnutrition is achieved by the mobilization of the tissue reserves of the mother whenever supplies of nutrients from the diet are inadequate. The effects of moderate degrees of maternal malnutrition on the outcome of a pregnancy are, therefore, not necessarily as harmful as might be expected, provided that the mother is well nourished before pregnancy. There can be no doubt, however, that severe and prolonged undernutrition during pregnancy increases the danger to the mother and to the infant.

There is a close relationship between birth weight and survival: below a certain weight, the lower the birth weight the greater is the chance of an infant being still-born or of dying within the first few days after birth. Nutrition, however, is only one factor influencing birth weight and there is no general agreement as to the extent to which nutrition during pregnancy influences birth weight in affluent societies. The effect of nutrition is certainly less than that of smoking which has a most profound effect on reducing birth weight.

In a population there is a close statistical relationship between the height of a mother and the birth weight of her child, i.e. short mothers tend to have small babies and vice versa. Clearly, the height of any individual is the product of both genetic and environmental factors but it is firmly established that nutrition during growth and development has a marked effect on mature height. It follows, therefore, that any stunting of growth brought about by poor nutrition during growth is likely to be associated with an increased risk of an unsuccessful pregnancy.

In most countries, women in the better-off sections of the community are more likely to give birth to strong, healthy infants than women in poor circumstances. In Britain, the rates of still-births and of infant mortality are much greater in social classes IV and V (partly skilled and unskilled occupations) than in social classes I and II (professional, managerial and senior administrative occupations). For example, in 1975/1976, infant mortality in the first year of life in the Yorkshire Regional Health Authority was 10 per 1000 in social classes I and II, 19 per 1000 in IV and 30 per 1000 in class V. A number of factors contribute to these huge differences and nutrition is one such factor, although its role has yet to be quantified.

There is good evidence that an inadequate intake of energy during pregnancy results in a reduction in the weight of infants at birth by something like 500 g but there is no reason to believe that poor maternal nutrition plays a significant part in the birth of pre-term infants of very low birth weight (less than 2 kg), although the infants themselves may be malnourished ('small-for-dates'). The WHO recommends the intake of an additional 1500 kJ day^{-1} during the second half of pregnancy but this assumes that physical activity continues to the same extent as before pregnancy. If physical activity declines, the energy requirement is also reduced.

The mean gain in weight during pregnancy is 12 kg of which c.4 kg is fat and women who seek to limit their weight gain by restricting energy intake run the risk of producing an infant lighter in weight than would otherwise be the case: furthermore, lactation potential may be impaired. The commonly accepted belief that excessive weight gain during pregnancy is undesirable relates particularly to the increase in weight due to excessive salt and water retention that occurs in 'pregnancy toxaemia' associated with hypertension, which has little to do with diet. It is accepted, however, that *excessive* deposition of fat to the point of obesity is to be avoided, since the extra fat may be difficult to lose after the baby is born, particularly if breast feeding is not adopted.

The additional amounts of protein required during pregnancy are surprisingly small and there is no reason to believe that any normal mixed diet will be limiting in protein provided that it is eaten in sufficient amounts to provide for energy requirements. There is some evidence that the utilization of dietary protein is more efficient in the pregnant than in the non-pregnant woman and this may explain why it is that women subsisting on diets that are really quite poor do not show signs of protein-deficiency during pregnancy. Nevertheless, if only as an insurance, all authorities recommend that pregnant women should have c. 10 g extra protein daily, an amount that can conveniently be provided by 300 ml (c. half a pint) of milk in countries where it is readily available.

The body of an average infant at birth contains c. 30 g calcium, most of which is accumulated during the last trimester, which implies a mean rate of storage of 330 mg day^{-1} during this period. During lactation 250–300 mg calcium day^{-1} may be secreted in the milk. Most national and international bodies recommend that the daily intake of calcium should be increased from 500 mg day^{-1} in the non-pregnant to 1200 mg day^{-1} in the pregnant and lactating woman. It is not difficult for these intakes to be attained by women in affluent societies, indeed, an extra 600 ml (c. one pint) of milk will provide the additional 700 mg calcium recommended, but it is virtually impossible for women in many developing countries to achieve these levels of intake. Indeed, it is doubtful if such high levels are necessary or even desirable, since there is reason to believe that women adapt to pregnancy by increasing the efficiency with which calcium is absorbed from the digestive tract. This is achieved by an increase in the plasma concentration of the active metabolite of vitamin D, the 1,25-dihydroxy derivative, probably under the influence of parathyroid hormone: prolactin may also be involved. The vitamin D-stimulated increase in calcium absorption persists into the lactation period.

Really low intakes of calcium that induce serious negative calcium balances during pregnancy and lactation can have serious effects on the mother. Whereas the skeletal reserves of calcium can be drawn upon for one or two pregnancies without impairing the strength of the bones, repeated pregnancies with little or no time between the weaning of the last infant and the birth of the next can result in severe osteoporosis due to loss of bone tissue.

The only other mineral that needs to be considered here is iron. It was noted earlier (p. 15) that absorption of iron from even the best diets may not be sufficient to prevent anaemia in young women and iron-deficiency anaemia is even more common in pregnant than in non-pregnant women, since the demands of the foetus for iron are substantial. Iron is required not only to support additional haemoglobin production but also to provide a liver store for the foetus during the last few weeks before birth. As a prophylactic measure, iron tablets are recommended throughout pregnancy for women who are anaemic and during the last trimester for all.

Women whose way of life does not allow them to obtain adequate amounts of vitamin D from exposure to sunlight (pp. 18–19) must be provided with a supplementary source of the vitamin during pregnancy if they are to avoid osteomalacia and if their infants are to be protected from rickets. Infants from mothers deficient in vitamin D may suffer from rickets at birth (congenital rickets) associated with hypocalcaemic tetany.

Folic acid is the only other vitamin deficiency which is widespread and in order to avoid the megaloblastic anaemia of pregnancy (pp. 16–17) a daily supplement of this vitamin is desirable.

Where deficiency of *any* vitamin is endemic, it goes without saying that pregnancy will increase requirements for that vitamin and increase the likelihood that symptoms of deficiency will appear in the mother, even if the foetus itself is protected by abstracting its requirements from the meagre supply available in the maternal blood.

During lactation, the requirements for energy and protein are somewhat higher than during the last trimester of pregnancy: the WHO recommends the intake of an additional 2.3 MJ energy and 17 g protein day^{-1} during lactation. Requirements for calcium are approximately the same for both physiological conditions but the requirements for iron are somewhat less in the nursing mother since milk is very low in iron. However, if a woman is prone to anaemia and if loss of blood during child-birth is great, the iron tablets should be continued. Although the foetus has priority over the mother for most vitamins, once the infant is born its priority is lost and the mammary gland does not appear able to concentrate vitamins from the blood. Thus, infantile beri-beri can occur in breast-fed infants, without the mother showing clinical signs of disease, presumably because the fast-growing infant has a higher requirement for thiamin than the mother.

Translating nutrient requirements for pregnancy and lactation into food, we arrive once more at the old prescription for a 'good mixed diet', which in western countries means a good mixture of milk and dairy products, margarine, fruit, vegetables, whole cereals and products derived from them, pulses, meat and fish in great variety, and not too much of any one.

5.2 Infants and children

For many thousands of years the only way to rear babies – if one excludes Romulus and Remus – was to suckle them at the breast and virtually all present day women have retained the ability to lactate abundantly. With the evolution of a social hierarchy, the upper social orders often employed members of the peasant classes to 'wet-nurse' their infants and thus arose the concept that it was not ladylike to feed babies at the breast and that breast-feeding was an activity suited to the lower social classes. The supply of wet-nurses must have been somewhat erratic and it was, no doubt, quite a break-through when techniques became available for the artificial feeding of infants using cows' milk.

The proportion of women breast-feeding their infants has varied from time to time in different societies according to economic circumstances, tradition, fashion, advertising and medical opinion. The swing to artificial feeding reached a peak in western Europe and North America in the 1960s when fewer than 20% of infants received breast milk.

If artificial feeding is best for the babies of fashionable ladies of the west and if the wealthy people in under-developed countries also feed their infants on the bottle, it is not surprising if poor peasant women in third world countries assume that artificial feeding must be best for their babies also, particularly if this belief is encouraged by large multi-coloured advertisements showing pictures of bonny babies sitting beside a tin of proprietary baby milk, and not actively discouraged by doctors and nurses. The result has been disastrous in terms of death and malnutrition. Whereas baby milk powders are first class products when made up with sterile water according to the manufacturers' directions under clean and hygienic conditions, they become a menace to health and even to life itself when prepared with contaminated water in unhygienic surroundings. Gastro-enteritis is the inevitable result. Furthermore, the milk is often made up at too low a concentration, either because the mother is illiterate and cannot read the instructions on the tin or because she cannot afford to prepare it at full strength. (Infant milks are products of high technology and are very expensive.) Feeding milk that is too dilute means that the intake of energy and protein is inadequate and protein-energy malnutrition is almost certain to develop.

Fortunately, the pendulum is now swinging in the other direction in western societies and mothers are now encouraged to breast-feed their infants for a few weeks at least. Many factors contributed to this change including the activities of enlightened pressure groups composed of women who felt passionately about the benefits of breast feeding to the infant in terms both of nutrition and of emotional development by bonding to their mother. Doctors, too, had become concerned about the increasing incidence of dietary allergies and of obesity in infants that had been artificially fed, although the latter problem was as much due to the early introduction of solid foods as to the feeding of milk formulae that were too concentrated. Although many more women are now breast-feeding in industrialized countries than in the recent past, the present situation gives no grounds for complacency. The biggest increase has been in middle-class women and in the poorer and less well educated sections of the community breast-feeding is a minority activity. In most parts of Europe, it is not considered decent to suckle an infant in public and changes in social attitudes are required if breast-feeding is to become a general practice. Women who go out to work have particular difficulties in breast-feeding and active members of the women's lib movement denounce breast-feeding as a sinister plot devised by man for the enslavement of women.

In purely nutritional terms, the benefits of breast-feeding are considerable; since human milk is the natural food for infants, its chemical composition in terms of fat, protein, carbohydrate, minerals and vitamins is ideally suited to their requirements for growth and development until solid feeding begins. Colostrum, the milk secreted during the first two days after birth, contains antibodies against a number of common infectious diseases: the anti-microbial agents lactoferrin (an iron-binding protein) and lysozyme are also present in breast milk. Even if mothers are unwilling to fully breast-feed, they could be strongly encouraged to give their infants the benefits of their colostrum: furthermore, breast-feeding confers a number of direct benefits to the mother. There can be no doubt that babies can be reared entirely successfully on the bottle and millions are so reared every year but bottle-feeding is more hazardous than breast-feeding and neonatal tetany (due to hypocalcaemia), dehydration (due to milk that is prepared in too concentrated a form) and gastro-enteritis (due to bacterial infections) are commoner in infants that are fed artificially. The ultimate decision on whether or not to breast-feed must be taken by the mother in the light of her own particular circumstances but doctors and nurses must accept the responsibility for acquainting all pregnant women with the advantages to both mother and infant of the natural method, which, fortunately, is much cheaper than the artificial system.

The main principle to observe in feeding infants 6–12 months of age, in addition to the basic principles that apply to individuals of all ages, is that the food offered must be highly digestible, which in practice means that the solid foods – cereals, vegetables, chicken, etc. – must be properly cooked, finely ground and free from lumps to give a product of porridge-like consistency. Custard, soft boiled egg yolk and mashed bananas are other favourite infant foods, and biscuits, rusks and fingers of bread and butter get them used to tackling more normal foods by using their teeth.

From about one year of age, the infants can be introduced to adult-type foods and before long they are eating the same meals as the family. However, toddlers have higher requirements for all nutrients and for energy than adults per kg body weight: the 'good mixed diet' that one hopes will be consumed by the parents and older children will ensure that adequate amounts of energy and of most nutrients are consumed and the extra requirements for protein, calcium and for a number of vitamins are most conveniently supplied by 600 ml (c. one pint) of milk daily, or its equivalent in protein from plant sources (pulses, nuts, etc.). Adequate exposure to sunlight will guard against a deficiency of vitamin D.

In school children aged 5–10, dietary requirements are not particularly exacting but a glass of milk a day is still recommended and so long as energy requirements are supplied dietary deficiencies are unlikely to arise. Under-nutrition during this period will, of course, impair growth in terms of both height and weight and over nutrition may lead to obesity. The great variation in the energy intake of children has been noted previously (p. 8). With the onset of puberty and its associated growth spurt, nutritional requirements increase once more and under-nutrition during adolescence will result in a reduction in adult height. Studies of the heights and weight of British school children have shown that both these indices of growth increased significantly during the fifty year period between 1910 and 1960. For example, the mean height of 13-year old Glasgow boys was 140 cm (55 inches) in 1920 and 152 cm (60 inches) in 1960: the corresponding weights were 34 kg (75 lb) and 43 kg (95 lb). There can be little doubt that better nutrition was primarily responsible for this improvement in growth but which particular nutrients were limiting growth in 1920 is not certain. Experiments carried out during the 1920s demonstrated the value of supplementary milk in increasing the height and weight of school children and for many years all children in Britain received one-third of a pint (200 ml) of milk free at school every day. Milk supplies generous amounts of energy, high quality protein, vitamins (particularly riboflavin) and calcium and all are important for growth.

Evidence from Japan suggests that calcium may be more important in influencing growth than had hitherto been recognized. Until 1950, the average daily intake of calcium in that country was c. 200 mg, far less than the RDI (500 mg) and a national programme for increasing the intake of this mineral was instituted at this time, as a result of which the mean daily calcium intake of children rose to c. 600 mg with only a slight increase in the intakes of energy and protein. There have been spectacular increases in the height of Japanese children in the past 30 years. In the two decades between 1950 and 1970 the mean height of 12 year old boys, for example, increased by 10 cm (4 inches) and the average young male adult is now significantly taller than his father and young women are almost always taller than their mothers.

The most serious problem of the nutrition of adolescents in Britain have already been discussed – anaemia (p. 15) and anorexia nervosa (pp. 11–12) in girls and rickets in children of Asian origin (pp. 18–19).

5.3 The elderly

Some people age sooner than others and it is a truism that people are as old as they feel. Nevertheless, it is an administrative convenience to be able to define old age and 65 is commonly accepted as the minimum age at which a person can be considered to be 'elderly'. Many old people lead an active life long after their retirement, playing golf, walking, gardening, etc., and for these people there is no reason to believe that their nutritional requirements differ significantly from the time when they were younger. For the majority of people, however, physical activity decreases in old age and for those who are more or less house-bound the decrease is substantial. It is with the nutrition of old people in this category that we shall mainly be concerned in this section.

Basal metabolic rate declines in the elderly, due to loss of lean-tissue mass and this decline together with the reduction in physical activity means that total energy expenditure and, therefore, energy requirements also decline. If therefore, energy intake continues at the same level as before, when they were younger, old people become obese and obesity is, in fact, quite common, particularly in elderly women. There is no reason to believe that requirements for protein, vitamins and minerals decline with age, however; indeed, they may even increase in particular cases, so that if a reduction in energy intake is achieved by eating less of all types of food, there is a possibility that nutritional deficiencies may develop. As in the case of weight-reducing diets (pp. 28–31), a reduced intake of energy should be achieved by cutting down on foods rich in sugar and fats, on 'empty calories', while maintaining the intake of protein-rich foods such as milk, cheese, eggs, meat, fish and pulses, which also supply important minerals and vitamins. The intake of dietary fibre should be maintained, if only to guard against constipation. The particular nutritional deficiencies from which elderly people are most likely to suffer are of vitamin C, vitamin D, folic acid, iron and potassium.

The nutrition of the elderly is inextricably mixed up with non-nutritional factors. The family situation greatly influences eating habits and elderly people living alone are very liable to eat a poor diet. Low income, poor cooking facilities and difficulties in shopping (fruit and vegetables, for example, are heavy to carry) can be all important in influencing diet. Digestive troubles and difficulties in chewing due to ill-fitting dentures also affect eating habits and all the problems mentioned above are magnified in old people suffering from medical conditions such as arthritis or cerebrovascular disease or from mental deterioration.

It is generally agreed that the most satisfactory way of ensuring that old people do not become malnourished is by providing them with a good mid-day meal, and luncheon clubs and meals-on-wheels do an excellent job in many communities. A major problem with all mass catering services is the inevitable loss of vitamin C that occurs when vegetables have to be cooked many hours before they are eaten and this vitamin may perhaps be provided most satisfactorily as orange or grapefruit juice. The diet cannot be relied upon to supply adequate amounts of vitamin D for elderly people who are house-bound and a daily supplement of the vitamin should therefore be given in the form of a pill. Nutritional anaemias in the elderly should be treated with iron and folic acid tablets.

Nutrition and longevity   There is no benefit to the individual and even less to society of living to a ripe old age unless mental and physical health are retained. To what extent does nutrition play a part in promoting longevity and in maintaining health in old age? It is not possible to answer this question with any certainty but a number of observations can usefully be made.

The number of very old people, centenarians, is greater in some populations than in others and the common feature of all communities in which the number of very old people is high, e.g. in mountainous areas of Ecuador, is that they are rural communities, the members of which occupy themselves in work on the land. Thus, it might be argued that clean, unpolluted air and hard physical work promote longevity. Life-span, like IQ, obesity, adult height and other physical and mental attributes, is the product of heredity and environment, of nature and nurture and of their inter-action, so that, in discussing the possible role of nutrition in slowing down the process of ageing it must be recognized that only part of the story is being considered. However, since it is not yet possible for human genes to be manipulated, this approach is wholly realistic.

The effect of diet on the life-span of experimental animals has been investigated by several different groups. The experimental results with laboratory animals are very consistent and all agree that restricting food intake in growing animals increases their longevity. In one particular experiment, rats were weaned at 28 d of age and from that time onwards fed either *ad libitum* or at 46% of this level of intake. The mean life-span of the male animals given unrestricted access to food was 802 d and of the restricted males 1005 d; the corresponding figures for females were 930 and 1294 d. In other experiments, energy restriction in middle life of rats fed *ad libitum* from weaning also prolonged life and increased the age at which malignant and degenerative diseases set in. These are precisely the types of disease to which elderly people are most prone, diseases such as cancer, arthritis and artery disease.

These studies certainly raise questions for the effects of nutrition on life span but they do not provide answers: men and women are not rats. Most people would find it difficult to accept the proposition that it is in the long-term interests of children to limit their rate of growth by restricting their food intake but a recommendation that food intake should be restricted to a level that permits normal growth without inducing obesity would be readily accepted, since this recommendation is consistent with evidence from other sources that obesity is to be avoided. The evidence from animal experiments that dietary restriction after growth has ceased extends the life span might be adduced in support of the view that over-eating should be discouraged and that is about as far as one can go.

Mortality statistics during the next fifty years should provide more concrete evidence of the link between nutrition and longevity in man, although the effects of other environmental factors such as the incidence of smoking and improvements in housing and sanitation and in combating illness by drugs and by other medical treatments, will also influence the statistics. Since the end of the Second World War, there have been great improvements in nutrition in western countries, particularly among the unskilled and semi-skilled classes. It will be interesting to see if these improvements are reflected in lower mortality rates for any particular diseases in the first few decades of the 21st century which the epidemiologists will be able to relate to infant and child nutrition. These improvements have already been reflected in increases in the height and weight of school-children in the 1950s and 1960s. However, it should not be forgotten that there were spectacular increases in the death rate from ischaemic heart disease in many affluent countries during the same twenty year period.

From time immemorial men have sought an 'elixir of youth', as fairy stories from many countries attest, and this search is now expressed in science fiction. Because orthodox science has been unable to come up with an answer – because there is no answer – the cranks and quacks of fringe medicine and pseudo-science have stepped in with their own prescriptions for extending life. Foremost among the magic potions they offer are the vitamins, and vitamin E is perhaps the elixir that is most commonly prescribed. Trace elements and various herbal extracts and other natural products are also offered for sale by the modern equivalent of witch doctors and medicine men who prey upon the ignorant and gullible seeking to delay the inevitable processes of senescence.

There will clearly be plenty of work for nutritionists to do for many years to come to determine what constitutes optimum nutrition for a long life span: meanwhile, we can say with absolute conviction that there is no pill or potion that will reverse or even slow down the ageing process and that the best nutritional advice that can be given is 'moderation in all things'. This message is not very exciting but people must understand there is no easy formula, no gimmicks, no magical diet that will ensure health and longevity and that the only answer is that good dietary habits should be implanted in youth and followed throughout life.

6 Concluding remarks

It is an article of faith among nutritionists that one of the essentials for good health is a good diet and during the last few years a number of official bodies from affluent countries have set down ways in which their national diets could be improved. Many of these reports were concerned particularly with making recommendations for reducing the risk of CHD but, by definition, a 'healthy' diet is one that minimizes the risk of all diseases and conditions with a strong nutritional component, including hypertension, diabetes and obesity as well as CHD and all diseases associated with mineral and vitamin deficiencies, so that one and the same set of recommendations applies to all normal people. It must be recognized, however, that people suffering from particular illnesses certainly do require special diets related to their particular disease.

An attempt has been made below to present a series of recommendations that represent the greatest possible measure of consensus between the various reports. Where no consensus emerges, the author's prejudices have prevailed! Although some of the reports are expressed in terms of national food goals or policies, the recommendations below are related to individuals.

1) Obesity, i.e. a body fat content of more than 35% in adults, should be avoided and individuals who are already obese should reduce their energy intake and/or increase their energy expenditure by taking more exercise in order to lose weight. Obesity in infants and children should also be avoided, primarily in order to inculcate good dietary habits from an early age, thus reducing the likelihood of adult obesity.

2) Total fat intake should not account for more than 35% of the total energy intake and this fat should be derived from as wide a variety of different plant and animal sources as possible to give a P:S ratio of 0.4 or more.

3) At least 50% of the total energy should be provided by carbohydrate, mainly in the form of starch and other complex carbohydrates derived from cereals, starchy roots and tubers and pulses.

4) Refined sugar from all sources should be restricted to a maximum of 100 g d^{-1}.

5) Dietary fibre is an important part of the diet but difficult to quantify. Provided that the target for total complex carbohydrates is achieved and provided that too high a proportion is not obtained from highly milled cereals, such as white flour, spaghetti and polished rice, there is no need to worry about dietary fibre.

6) Fruit and vegetables should be included in at least one meal per day and the consumption of raw fruit and vegetables (apples, oranges, tomatoes, lettuce, cabbage, carrots, etc.) should be encouraged.

7) The maximum daily consumption of salt that is desirable is 5 g.

8) Infants should be breast-fed whenever possible.

Final note: There are no bad foods, only bad diets.

Further Reading

ALLEYNE, G. A. O., HAY, R. W., PICON, D. I., STANFIELD, J. P. and WHITEHEAD, R. G. (1977). *Protein-Energy Malnutrition*. Edward Arnold, London.

AYKROYD, W. R. (1974). *The Conquest of Famine*. Chatto and Windus, London.

AYLWARD, F. and JUL, M. (1975). *Protein and Nutrition Policy in Low-Income Countries*. Charles Knight, London and Tonbridge.

BENDER, A. E. (1975). *Dictionary of Nutrition and Food Technology*, 4th edn. Newnes-Butterworth, London.

BENDER, A. E. (1975). *The Facts of Food*. Oxford University Press, Oxford.

DAVIDSON, S., PASSMORE, R., BROCK, J. F. and TRUSWELL, A. S. (1979). *Human Nutrition and Dietetics*, 7th edn. Churchill Livingstone, Edinburgh, London and New York.

DOBBING, J. (1981). *Maternal Nutrition in Pregnancy: Eating for Two?* Academic Press, London.

FOOD AND AGRICULTURE ORGANISATION OF THE UNITED NATIONS (1973). *Energy and Protein Requirements*. FAO Nutrition Report series No. 52, Rome.

GARROW, J. S. (1978). *Energy Balance and Obesity in Man*, 2nd edn. North Holland/Elsevier, Amsterdam, London and New York.

HMSO (1976). *Manual of Nutrition*, 8th edn. London.

HMSO (1974). *Food and Nutrition Research*. London and Elsevier Scientific Publishing Company, Amsterdam and New York.

JARRETT, R. J. (Ed.) (1979). *Nutrition and Disease*. Croom Helm, London.

McLAREN, D. S. (1981). *Nutrition and its Disorders*, 3rd edn. Churchill Livingstone, Edinburgh and London.

MOTTRAM, V. H. (1976). *Human Nutrition*, 2nd edn. Edward Arnold, London.

OLSON, R. A. (Ed.) (1975). *Protein-Calorie Malnutrition*. Academic Press, London.

PAUL, A. A. and SOUTHGATE, D. A. T. (1978) McCance and Widdowson's *The Composition of Foods*, 4th edn. HMSO, London.

PYKE, M. (1970). *Man and Food*. Weidenfeld and Nicolson, London.

ROBSON, J. R. K. (1972). *Malnutrition* (2 vols). Gordon and Breach, New York.

TAYLOR, T. G. (Ed.) (1979). *The Importance of Vitamins to Human Health*. MTP Press, Lancaster.

WINICK, M. (1976). *Malnutrition and Brain Development*. Oxford University Press, Oxford.

YUDKIN, J. (Ed.) (1978). *Diet of Man: Needs and Wants*. Applied Science Publishers, London.

Index